Train Smarter, Not Harder

fitness guide for executives and desk jockeys

By Traci Riley
©Traci Trainer Fitness, LLC

Library of Congress Cataloging in Publication Data

Riley, Traci G.
 Train Smarter, Not Harder fitness guide for executives and desk jockeys
 1. Self-publishing

ISBN # 1438214685

Train Smarter, Not Harder fitness guide for executives and desk jockeys

Cover photo and design by photographer Kim Lemaire

Cover Model: Kim Ruiz

Logo Design by Laurie Bend

Anatomical Illustrations: Real Bodywork @ www.realbodywork.com

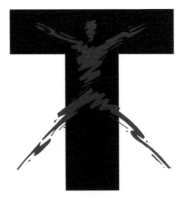

FORWARD

You have been caught! I caught you! Stand up straight! Legs uncrossed! Feet flat on the floor! Shoulders back! Head up! Nope, we aren't back in grade school class, but Ms. Jones may have had your best interest in mind when correcting your posture "back in the day."

When was the last time you or Ms. Jones focused on your posture, not to mention the rest of your body? Though, it may be many moons later, you've taken a grand first step towards physical fitness success, injury prevention, and wellness by reading past this book's cover. Start your goal-oriented, self-directed fitness plan today with the help of Traci Riley's innovative and proven techniques. By using her approach, you will improve your overall physical and mental health, as well as enhance your lifestyle.

Michael J. Wheeler, PT, DPT, ATC

Executive Endorsements

… a skillful assessor of the client's condition and has a knack for recommending the right program.

70-year-old Professor

… not only is she knowledgeable in all areas of fitness, she has a tremendous understanding of the body and the physical therapy aspects of a proper training program.

Colonel, U.S. Marine Corps

… expand the sphere of influence of the fitness trainer, Traci Riley, to every command leadership venue feasible. Mrs. Riley embodies the passion and junior officer spirit essential to every successful wardroom, ready room, and mess.

Captain, U.S. Navy

… I am a successful climber of Kilimanjaro; in fact I was in better shape for this activity than all 26 people who climbed – rivaled only by a 25-year-old.

63-year-old Senior Executive

… fitness strategies and tips offered specifically for individuals leading busy and stressful lives have already been helpful. Traci instilled in the class that health is a personal responsibility and empowered us to take charge.

Admiral, U.S. Navy

… I am now one of your exercise apostles! I have felt so much better and frankly my wife has noticed that I am not so thick in the waist, I am no longer the "hamster in the wheel."

Retired Lt. Colonel, U.S. Marine Corps

… You have helped me increase my lean body mass, improve my flexibility, as well as trim 43 seconds off my running time. I attribute this to increased flexibility and your cardio training.

Major, U.S. Marine Corps

… I always seemed to hit a plateau but after working with Traci; I am amazed by the very noticeable changes in my body in just five weeks!

40-year-old female Professional

… You taught me how to exercise smart to build muscle to burn more calories when I worked out and in four months, I have lost 15 lbs and 10 ½ inches and my husband thinks I am hot. Thanks, I couldn't have done it without you.

40-year-old Senior Executive

Dedicated to my husband, Sean, who motivates me to stay fit,
my daughters Rebecca & Seanna who inspire me to live a healthy lifestyle,
and my mother, Rebecca, who is living proof that diet, exercise,
and managing stress are the keys to a happier, healthier life!

Contents

Introduction

It's time to learn exercises and routines that not only help you reach your fitness goals, but are also fun and challenging. I will teach you how to **be your own personal trainer**! I will take you step by step through the process of an initial assessment. You will learn how to assess your current fitness level, set attainable goals, and develop your own personalized exercise program.

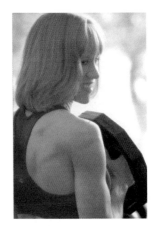

If you don't like going to the gym, no problem; try the "No Gym Required" workout. If you are always on the go, learn exercises you can do anywhere. Maximize caloric burn by doing in 10 minutes what it takes most others an hour to do. If you are a weekend warrior, learn how to reduce and avoid your chances of injury. If you are saddled with pain, become pain-free by correcting your posture, using proper exercise form, and choosing the right stretches and exercises for you.

I have over a decade of educational experience enriching people's lives through public, private, and governmental education programs and received my Personal Trainer accreditation from the National Academy of Sports Medicine. My results-driven programs led the Naval Post-Graduate School in Monterey, CA, to invite me to teach their strength, core, and biomechanics classes, as well as become their on-site personal trainer. I worked exclusively with individual clients, training hundreds of people, ranging in age from 9 to 94.

Over 98 percent of my clients came to me either in pain or with pre-existing injuries they had sustained during their lifetimes. I will share with you what I learned about injury prevention while working as a physical therapy aide, so that you may be able to avoid any future needs for your own physical therapy. I will share with you what I learned about physical rehabilitation as well, so that you may get relief from any aches or pains that you already have.

I currently run an effective health and wellness program for the Navy leadership through the Navy's Executive Learning Office. The program involves lecturing and demonstrating all the principles you will read in this book to admirals and other Navy senior leaders.

This intense, almost full-time experience with fitness and physical therapy has been enormously rewarding and exciting. It is truly a euphoric moment when you realize you have found your niche in your professional life. This moment came for me when I received a letter of recommendation written by a respected, retired Navy admiral, part of which stated: "She instills a motivation for long-term, healthy lifestyle changes. Her approach provides life-transforming knowledge and fitness-training tips. Her competence is off the chart! I appreciate her passionate and caring attitude; she's one of the best – if not the best. Her fitness program was a very personalized and practical way to improve health, increase fitness, and reduce stress."

Reading this was the highlight of my career, because my goal with all my clients is to help them develop long-term healthy lifestyle changes. I have always taken great pride in my husband's career as a Marine; however, working so closely with the Navy has given me, personally, the chance to make a difference in the lives of those who sacrifice so much for this country. This book is providing me yet another unique opportunity – to share with *you* the successful techniques and programs that have worked for me and so many others.

Your exercise program should relieve stress, not create it. Try the "20 Minute Stress Reliever Routine." Avoid hitting a plateau and exercising like a hamster in a wheel. Instead, use my guidelines for choosing just the right exercises for you from those I have provided in this book. You will be able to create several dynamic warm-ups and exercise programs that will be designed specifically for you and your specific needs and limitations. This book is designed to motivate you by seeing your own results and to keep you challenged for optimal performance and health. Keep in mind that before you begin any fitness program you should consult with your physician.

Chapter One: How Fit Are You?
Assessing your waist, posture, and diet

I always have my clients fill out a PAR-Q before I even meet with them. A PAR-Q is a basic questionnaire that personal trainers use to get a baseline fitness level of a potential client. You will use the same PAR-Q to get your baseline fitness level. Even if you are already an avid exerciser it is important that you assess your waist, posture, and diet. Your waist measurement could be an indication of potential health risks and will help you set attainable goals. Assessing your current posture helps you understand how it affects the way you sit, stand, exercise, and sleep. Correcting your posture will help you exercise with proper form, prevent injuries, and live a more pain-free life. Taking a good look at your diet allows you to see where you can make small changes that could potentially improve your mood, energy levels, sleep cycle, and overall health.

Unlike most personal trainers who use a weight scale or body mass index scale (BMI) to set goals and track a client's progress, I prefer a tape measure. Weight can fluctuate from day-to-day and a client's motivation can be negatively affected if the number that appears on the scale is not what they were hoping for. Clients who use the BMI scale, which provides a range of acceptable weights for

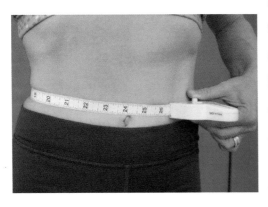

an individual, are sometimes confused as to what their weight should be. The circumference of your waist is not only important to your confidence level, self-esteem, and the way your body physically appears to you and others; it also determines potential health risks. Ideally a woman's waist should measure 32 ½ inches and a man's should measure 35 inches. Women with waists measuring more than 35 inches and men with waists measuring more than 40 inches have a higher risk of heart disease, diabetes, and other health problems.

The first order of business is to measure your waist with your clothes off (taking this measurement over your clothes will give you an inaccurate reading). Place the tape around your waist, starting and ending at your belly button, while using your abdomen muscles to pull your belly button back toward your spine as if being pulled by a string. Record your waist measurement so that you will be able to track your progress. You *will* make progress. And seeing the number drop may be all the motivation you need to get fit and healthy.

You can exercise religiously an hour a day, but if you are consuming too many calories the other 23 hours, there isn't anything anyone can do to help you. There is only one way to find out what you are truly eating and it requires a little discipline on your part. Keep a log of everything you put in your mouth for nine days. I mean *everything*! Even if you grab a piece of candy or a mint from someone's desk at work, log it. It is important that you don't alter what you normally eat in order to have an accurate account of your habits. When the log is complete, circle all of the vegetables, underline all of the fruit, and highlight the one item you see over and over again. Now ask yourself the following questions:

-How many vegetable servings are listed? (Hopefully, there are *some* vegetables listed. Many times a client's log doesn't have any vegetables listed, other than in a Chinese stir-fry!)

-Do I always eat the same vegetable or is there a variety?

-How many fruit servings are listed?

-Is there a rainbow of fruits or does the same fruit appear over and over again? (Most of the time only bananas are listed on a client's log; probably because they are so convenient to eat.)

-What kind of snacks am I eating and what is their caloric content? (Snacks should be kept between 100-125 calories.)

-Do I eat three small meals a day with two snacks? (Most people skip breakfast, gorge at lunch, and eat a large, late dinner.)

-What beverages am I consuming and what is their calorie content? (Most people consume far too many liquid calories.)

-Do I have a reoccurring item that is not so healthy? (For example: mocha frappuccino lattes, candy, chips or alcohol.)

-Do I take a vitamin supplement?

Most people who take this task seriously are shocked by the results. But statistically, they reach their goals faster. The results give you an accurate depiction of your diet and a good place to start setting goals for yourself. You don't need a registered dietitian to tell you that a strawberry frappuccino and apple fritter are not the best choices for breakfast. Attempting a perfect diet from this point on will set you up to fail. Instead, decide on one or two changes you can make (for example: drink more water, eat dark chocolate instead of milk chocolate, cook with less salt, trade Skippy® for a natural peanut butter, or take one less sugar when ordering coffee). After about a month, when you have successfully made these changes, make one or two more. Every month your diet will improve as you establish new habits while making healthier choices.

Ok, you survived the task of measuring your waist, have beaten yourself up enough concerning your diet, now it's time to assess your body's frame. You may think you look engaged in conversation with a colleague while standing with your arms folded in front of you and resting them on your protruding belly; or authoritative while leaning to one side with your hand on your hip. In actuality, you are doing long-term damage to your body's frame. You continue to damage your frame throughout the day by sitting hunched over a desk or in a long meeting with your legs crossed the same way every time or if you travel by air, you will inevitably be shoved into an airplane seat not big enough for a child. You may make sure you have perfect form while exercising – and by all means you should – but your habits the rest of the day could do you in.

Poor posture leads to muscle imbalances that lead to chronic pain, joint injuries, and, quite possibly, a moment in your life where you might be the person yelling, "Help, I've fallen and I can't get up!" (FYI: Hip fractures are the leading cause of death in elderly people.) It is just as important to maintain good posture while sitting and standing throughout the day as it is to have good form when you exercise or a proper gait while walking and proper stride when running. Keep in mind that your muscles pull your bones into place. This is not rocket science. If your muscles are imbalanced, they will pull your bones out of balance.

I want you to perform a simple squat assessment that will give you valuable information specific to your frame. This assessment will tell you how your body is moving, even when you aren't paying attention. What you see will determine what stretches and exercises are needed, if any, to correct your posture and maintain a healthy frame. The goal here is to stretch the muscles that are tight and strengthen the muscles that are weak. By doing so, your muscles will pull your bones into proper alignment. You should perform the squat assessment every four weeks to check your progress and to help you choose your stretches and exercises for the next workout plan.

Squat Assessment: Facing a mirror, stand with your feet hip width apart and toes pointed straight ahead. Now, lift your arms up so that they are parallel with your ears, palms facing the mirror. Perform ten squats while watching yourself closely as you move. Record what you see on the PAR-Q provided. (It is also helpful to ask a partner to watch you.) You are looking to see if your:

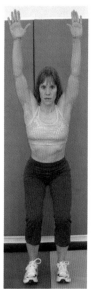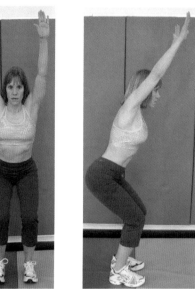

- feet externally rotate (toes point away from your body)
- heels come up off the floor
- knees go out as if you are bow-legged or in as if you are knock-kneed
- hips shift to one side.

Now turn to the side and perform ten more squats. Record what you see on the PAR-Q provided. You should be looking to see if your:

- back arches to the point that your butt sticks out
- back rounds to the point that your butt tucks under, like a dog being scolded
- arms fall forward and do not stay in alignment with your ears
- head falls forward

Bring your arms down and place your hands on your hips. Perform a squat standing on only one leg. Keep one foot off the ground, but close enough to tap down to maintain your balance, if necessary.

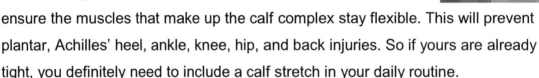

You may notice during this assessment that your balance is either poor or non-existent. Don't fret, I will teach you the balance exercises necessary to keep you from being "that person who fell and couldn't get back up." It doesn't matter which leg you balance on first, because you will need to perform the single leg squat assessment on each leg. Look for the same movements as before. They may be more exaggerated now that you are on one leg. This will help you determine if your results from the first assessment were correct.

If you noted that your toes pointed outward away from your body or that your heels rose off the floor, it means that your calves are tight. Every routine should include a calf stretch to ensure the muscles that make up the calf complex stay flexible. This will prevent plantar, Achilles' heel, ankle, knee, hip, and back injuries. So if yours are already tight, you definitely need to include a calf stretch in your daily routine.

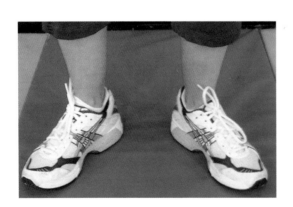 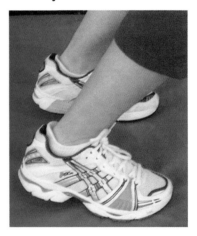

If you noted that your knees go out as if bow-legged (usually more of a problem for men), your body is telling you that the muscles in the back of your legs and your butt are tight; specifically, the bicep femoris and piriformis. If your knees tried to touch as if knock-kneed, the muscles on the insides of your legs, otherwise known as the adductors, are tight and your hip muscles weak.

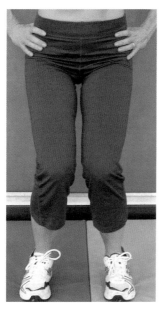 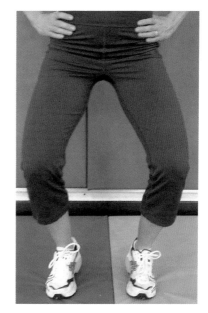

If you moved with your butt tucked under, the muscles in the back and inside of your legs are tight. If you stuck your butt out and appeared sway-backed; then the muscles located in front of your body where the hips join the leg (hip flexors), and the back muscles that run parallel to the spine, are tight. This is probably the result of sitting for long periods of time and/or not stretching properly after you exercise.

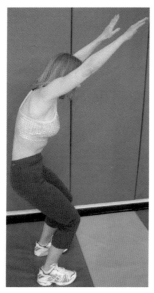 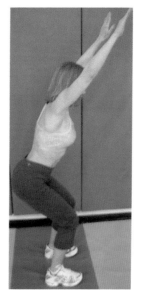

If your hips shifted to one side, then the adductor muscles (inside your thigh) on the same side as the shift, and the piriformis (your butt) on the opposite side of the shift, are tight. (Think: Do you find yourself standing with your hip protruding out to one side and your hand resting on your hip?)

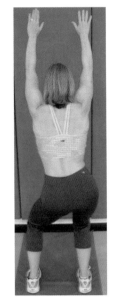

If your hands fell forward and you struggled to keep your arms in line with your ears, then your chest muscles, otherwise known as your pecs, are tight. Tight pecs are just as common with desk jockeys as with weightlifters. If you are slumped over a computer all day, your pecs will get tight while your shoulders and upper back muscles get overstretched and weak. Did you notice that your head fell forward? If so, your levator scapula and scalene muscles are also weak and elongated. This posture will ensure that your cervical spine (neck) gets out of alignment trying to support your heavy head; and give you all sorts of problems, such as headaches and unattractive, painful humps at the base of your neck.

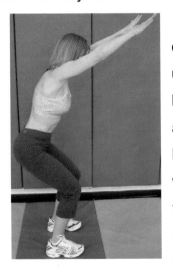

Also, using a mouse with the same arm every time can make one pec tighter than the other. Most people use the right shoulder more than the left, resulting in long-term imbalances in the shoulder girdle. Get up and go look in the mirror. Do both of your shoulders look the same or does one appear to be rolled forward with a deep crevice where the chest meets the arm at the base of the shoulder? I call this "mouse arm." If you have "mouse arm" you will need to do pec stretches more often on this arm, and if possible, switch hands every now and then when using the mouse. We will discuss in detail how you will apply this information in chapters four and six.

Traci Trainer Physical Assesment Readiness Questionnaire (PAR-Q)

train smarter not harder

Starting Waist Measurement: _____
Does your body do the following during squat assessment?

Observable imbalance indicators	Two- Legged Squat		Single Leg Squat	
	Yes	No	Yes	No
feet externally rotate				
heels come up off the floor				
knees turn in (knock-kneed)				
knees bow out				
hips shift to the right or left				
back arches with butt protruding				
lower back rounds (i.e. cowering dog)				
arms fall forward not aligned with ears				
head and chin fall forward				

What are your specific goals?

_____

_____

_____

Where will you work out? _____

Will you work out with someone or go it alone? _____

What days can you work out? _____

How long do you have to work out each day? _____

Recreational activities:

_____

_____

Sports: _____

Injuries: _____

Surgeries: _____

Current Pain or any pre-existing conditions:

_____

_____

Chapter Two: Who Are You?
Setting Attainable Goals

Knowing where to start can be the toughest job when making the decision to take better care of yourself. Even if you are a health nut, knowing what you could do to be healthier – or what new goal to set next – can be a real problem. If it weren't a major issue Americans wouldn't be facing a growing obesity epidemic today. Every year from mid-December through mid- January, countless TV programs inform people of ways to stick to their New Year's resolutions. January through March, gyms become overcrowded with people who have made "getting fit" their New Year's resolution. By the end of March, the majority will have hit a plateau and given up their resolution rather than making a goal-directed change in their routine which would have allowed them to bust through their plateau with the necessary motivation to continue their program. When making fitness goals, most people are simply not realistic. Most underestimate their physical capabilities and overestimate what they are willing to do to reach their goals.

Goals should:

-be specific

-be attainable

-be somewhat enjoyable

-fit into your daily lifestyle

-be measureable and recorded

You can't just say, "I want to be healthy," show up at the gym, and expect to know what to do. You must have a plan. By being specific ("I want to run the St. Patty's Day 5K race in March"), you can actually design a program, or have a fitness professional design a program, that will help you reach your goal.

Be realistic, if you are 100 pounds overweight and want to run the 5K in a month, this goal would probably not be attainable. By setting attainable, realistic goals you increase your chances of success. Actually running the 5K race allows you to measure and record reaching your goal. If you would rather eat nails than run, understand that the training required to run a 5K would neither be enjoyable nor fit your daily lifestyle. There are so many great ways to exercise it is unnecessary to choose activities you dislike doing.

First, you need to choose where you like to exercise. Whether it is at home, a gym, outside, or a combination of places, the location may limit your choices when designing your program. Determine if you are going to take exercise classes, work out with a partner, go it alone, or a combination thereof. Next, determine what days you have available to exercise and how much time you can allocate on each given day. It would be optimal if you could allocate five days a week to exercise, spending three days a week on resistance training and two days on cardio; but it may not be realistic. You might only have ten minutes a day to exercise; therefore, you will need to optimize those ten minutes. Don't be the person who says, "Well I can't do 30 minutes so I'll just skip today". Even if you only have five minutes to stretch, do so.

Next, make a list of exercises, sports, or recreational activities you enjoy. You will design your exercise routine around these activities, as well as choose exercises to improve your skills thus making them more enjoyable. If you like to play golf, then allot time in your exercise routine for golf. In addition, perform exercises that will help take strokes off your game or increase your driving distance and, at the same time, reduce your risk of injury.

The key to sticking with an exercise program is choosing the right place, time, and activity by which to get started. If you have the time, are doing something you like to do, and are comfortable with your surroundings, you will eventually establish a routine because the benefits will become obvious and the results will keep you going. It takes 30 days to create a habit, but only three days to break one. Take the next 30 days to "create the habit of living healthy."

Once you have determined:

    -where you will work out

    -if you will work out with someone or go it alone

    -when you will work out and for how long

    -what recreational activities or sports will be included

    -your specific, attainable, goal- record it on the PAR-Q provided.

Chapter Three: Everything Hurts
Becoming Pain-Free

I hear it constantly: "I can't exercise, my _____ hurts too much." I've got news for you. Your _____ will get worse, and take the rest of you down with it, if you don't start moving. At age 11 I was diagnosed with scoliosis; age 23, whiplash; age 36, an acute injury to my thoracic spine; and age 38 two ligament tears in my right ankle. In each case, I used exercise to rehabilitate the injured area. I continue to live pain-free by using exercise to stay strong and flexible.

Last December, I was performing plyometric lateral jumps using a bench at the gym, when my shoelaces came loose. I lost my balance; fell onto a nearby multipurpose bench, landing on a metal strip directly between T9 and T10 – the thoracic vertebrae in the middle of my back. I experienced some pain, but continued to work out, thinking my ego had sustained more of an injury than my back.

Within ten minutes I realized I was bleeding and immediately went to the emergency room. After waiting for more than two hours, all the time wondering what a personal trainer does if she is unable work out, I was taken to X-ray. During the X-ray I panicked at the thought of no longer being physically capable of doing my job. It is one thing if you decide to leave a job because you want to; but quite another to discover you will no longer be able to do a job you love because your health won't allow it.

The Boniva commercial kept playing in my mind and I heard, over and over, Sally Field say, "I have one life and one body to live it in, so I take care of myself." I cannot begin to tell you how elated I was to hear the doctor say the words, "Well, there are no spine fractures. You have sustained only bruised muscles." I breathed a sigh of relief.

The doctor smiled and said, "Here, take this," and shoved a tiny blue pill and Dixie cup of water at me. A doctor's solution almost always includes anti-inflammatory meds or pain relievers. When I finally awoke, late afternoon the next day, I felt like I had been hit by a truck. My vision was blurry, my mouth was dry, and I was totally exhausted. I discovered that the little blue pill was Valium and that I had been given a 10-day supply.

Considering that, at the time, I was working two jobs and had two children to take care of; I couldn't spend the next ten days drooling all over myself. I decided not to take the pills and went back to the gym with every intention of working slowly back up to my previous training level. I was working as a physical therapy aide at the time, so I asked one of the therapists how I could get safely back into my exercise program. After a thorough examination, the therapist suggested that I take the anti-inflammatory medication but avoid taking the Valium if possible. He informed me that the worst thing I could do was allow my joints to stiffen. He advised me to exercise using good form and in a pain-free range of motion rather than lie in bed.

While researching exercises for the middle back, I came upon thoracic extensions. They ended up being the miracle cure for my injured back. I worked up to two sets of fifteen reps, three times per week, with a 24-hour rest period in between. The combination of this therapeutic exercise with an erector spinae stretch had me back to my normal lifting routine in three days.

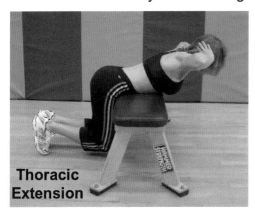
Thoracic Extension

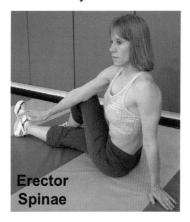
Erector Spinae

The key to my success was:

    -seeking and taking the advice of a trusted professional

    -finding the right exercise to strengthen the weakened, injured muscles

    -making sure the exercise could be performed in a pain-free range of motion

    -keeping the joints moving and the muscles surrounding the joints flexible

    -recognizing my weaknesses and not pushing my limits

Performing exercises in a pain-free range of motion is good advice for anyone, even if they aren't injured. I do not believe in the philosophy, "no pain, no gain." Pain is your body's way of communicating with you. If you ever experience a stabbing pain when performing an exercise, stop and correct your form. If the pain persists, the exercise you are performing may not be right for you. However, a burning sensation in the muscle toward the end of a set means you are achieving muscle fatigue, which is considered a "good" pain when exercising.

What do I mean by knowing your strengths but, more importantly, knowing your weaknesses? Whether you sustained an injury in high school or last week, each injury is a weak link you should take into account when performing exercises. As I said earlier, I was diagnosed with scoliosis at age 11. I actually have three curvatures, each located in a different section of my spine. The spine is broken down into three sections: cervical (neck), thoracic (middle back), and lumbar (lower back).

My largest curve is located in the thoracic section, the same one I injured last December. Now you know why I was so panicked. It is also the curve that caused me the most pain as a teenager. It hurt when I stood up, sat down, lay in bed, or moved. I tried heating pads, ice packs, Motrin, and massage therapy. Nothing seemed to work. Doctors tried topical rubs, medications, and painful injections – leaving spine surgery as my only option. No big deal! They just wanted to shove a metal rod up my spine. On the bright side, it could make me a few inches taller. This was not exactly great news for a high-school senior who was looking forward to college.

I opted not to have surgery; but that didn't mean I was ready to live my life in constant pain. I took up weight lifting, intending to keep my body in the best shape possible. Soon my back pain became manageable and remained so for the remainder of high school.

Unfortunately, in college the only exercise I got was when I danced. I worked two jobs that required standing eight hours straight, and spent the rest of my day sitting in class. This lifestyle played havoc with my back.

Then, in less than a year, I fell in love and married a Marine. We moved to Cherry Point, N.C. I took a job teaching preschool and learned that lifting children wasn't any easier on my back than sitting all day. After being transferred to Okinawa, I sustained a neck and shoulder injury in a car crash.

It was at this time that my husband took up serious weightlifting which was a turning point in my life. At age 23, I realized that while a lifestyle of eating Snickers and watching movies would be dreamy, it was not realistic. My neck, shoulder, and back were in constant pain and my husband was dreaming of baby number two. Trust me when I say a woman needs to be fit *before* deciding to get pregnant. I worked exercise back into my schedule, making it just as important in my daily routine as brushing my teeth. I no longer take any form of pain or anti-inflammatory medication, and I have been almost completely pain-free since that day. I attribute this solely to exercise. And if I can do it, so can you!

Now when I choose exercises, I first take into account my pre-existing injuries which include my neck, back, right shoulder, and right ankle.

Where did the ankle come into play, you ask? I had been asked to interview with the USMC Expeditionary Warfare School at Quantico who was evaluating my fitness program to see if it would benefit the Marines attending the school. My husband insisted that I run the Combat Endurance Course at Quantico to get an idea of what Marines must physically be able to do. I agreed, because this made sense, and I like to challenge myself once a year to do something I have never done before. What a fool!

Several times, while standing on a log nine feet above the ground praying I wouldn't fall and kill myself, I thought, "You are almost 40! What are you trying to prove?"

Believe it or not, I survived the logs and ropes only to be taken down by a tree stump at mile marker number four. As I fell, screaming in pain, I realized I still had two miles left to complete the course. My husband wanted to carry me over his shoulder for the remainder of the course, but my ego wouldn't allow it. I ran the last two miles, with two torn ligaments in my ankle. It required six months for a full recovery.

After an MRI and a consultation with an orthopedic surgeon, I began icing my ankle for 15 minutes every two hours, and exercised with a Thera-Band® to increase strength and range of motion. After just two days using these techniques I was jumping rope for 10 minutes, lifting weights, and preparing for my next fitness conference.

Combining my own experiences with the data collected for over three years while training executives, I learned the most common physical complaints are associated with the neck, shoulder, back, knee, and foot. I have found that most of the executives I work with get relief from this pain through exercise and stretching techniques. I have even been told that not only did their pain subside, but they were able to cancel surgery appointments and resume activities they previously had been unable to do. Therefore I am including in this book, common injuries that are associated with these aches and pains. Prepare yourself for a quick, but necessary anatomy lesson. I promise to keep it as brief as possible. Let's start at the feet and work our way up!

<u>Plantar Fasciitis, Heel Spurs, Heel Pain</u>

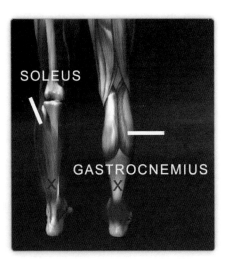

Plantar Fasciitis is the most common cause of heel pain. It occurs when the long, fibrous plantar fascia ligament along the bottom of the foot develops tears. Most people feel a burning, stabbing, or aching pain in the heel. Pain usually occurs after long periods of standing, sitting, or during/after physical activity.

Wearing shoes that do not fit properly or provide inadequate support and cushioning can damage the plantar ligament. When you exercise in ill-fitting shoes, your weight is not distributed properly. This puts significant stress on the ligament. Sports-related activities like running, jumping, and even regular exercise routines – or being overweight – place repetitive, excessive stress on the ligament. This causes tears that can result in mild to severe pain. Having flat feet, high arches, over pronation, or an abnormal gait pattern (from the way in which the foot strikes the ground through the way it leaves the ground), can overload the ligament, which can result in tears and inflammation as well.

Heel Spurs are pointed, bony fragments that stem from the heel bone, put pressure on sensitive tissue and nerves, and cause pain with every step. The pointed growths of bone develop when the plantar fascia ligament is repetitively pulled away from the heel bone. Heel spurs can develop alone or in conjunction with plantar fasciitis.

The Achilles tendon runs vertically up from the heel towards the ankle and knee. If pain is felt behind the heel, it could be a sign of **Achilles tendonitis**. It may swell, look red, or feel warm to the touch.

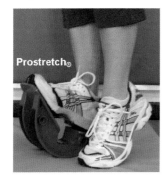

To avoid injuries in your ankles and feet you need to maintain a healthy weight, wear shoes that fit well and replace them every six to eight months, and make sure that your calf muscles are strong and flexible enough to move with a good range motion. Picture your calf muscle, which stretches from your heel to your knee, with limited range of motion because it is tight and weak. When you try to move, your calf muscle will be unable to perform the requested task, forcing it to recruit other muscles attached to your knees or ankles, thereby increasing the risk of causing an injury to one or both of the joints. To avoid injury I use a Medidyne Prostretch® to protect my plantar ligaments while stretching my calf muscles.

Knee Injuries

Knee surgeries and nagging knee pain aren't just a problem for athletes. Everyone, young and old, visits their doctors with common knee ailments. Sometimes when young people experience a growth spurt, their muscles and tendons don't grow as fast as their bones. When this happens the hamstrings and quads become tight and pull the knee out of good postural alignment. For middle-aged to older adults, knee problems are usually the result of weight gain, overuse, inflexibility, a sedentary lifestyle or combination thereof. Although you may not be able to avoid every knee problem, there are stretches and exercises you can do to provide your knees a little insurance.

The **vastus medialis oblique** muscle (VMO) is supposed to stabilize the patella (kneecap), medially and laterally with the help from the vastus lateralis muscle. When your VMO is strong it keeps your patella in its patellar groove. When weak, your patella can move into an abnormal position, causing pain and your knee joint to become unstable. If your quadriceps (the muscle located in the front of your upper thigh) are weak, avoid leg

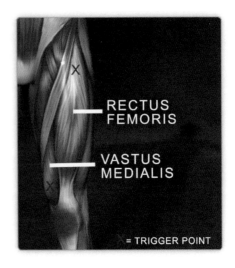

extensions if they cause pain. Instead, perform body-weight squats, single leg squats, quad sets, and other knee stabilizer exercises to strengthen them. Your hip muscles also aid in stabilizing your knee, so add side-lying leg raises to your workout. It is also important to keep your hamstrings, quads, calves and glute muscles stretched.

The **menisci** (cartilage), located between the tibia and femur, also help stabilize your knee by functioning as shock absorbers. If the menisci are torn from an overuse or impact injury, the knee may become inflamed and painful. An MRI would be necessary to positively detect a tear, as well as determine if treatment should consist of anti-inflammatory medications, icing and aggressive rehabilitation, or if it will require arthroscopic surgery. To avoid damage to the menisci, keep the musculature that surrounds your knee strong and flexible. Use proper landing mechanics when performing plyometric exercises (which will reduce the amount of force the menisci needs to absorb during landing), stay hydrated, and maintain a healthy weight.

Iliotibial Band (ITB) Syndrome is one of the leading causes of lateral knee pain in runners and women. This fascia band is a gristle-like material which runs the length of the outer thigh, starting at the hip and inserting below the knee. It is difficult to stretch and gets restricted blood flow, making it equally difficult to heal if it becomes aggravated and inflamed. When you run, the band should stabilize your

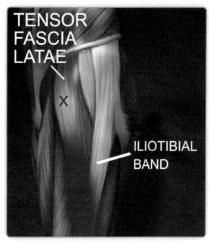

knee as it moves from behind the lateral condyle towards the front of the knee during your stride. Many women suffer ITB Syndrome because the position of their hips causes their legs to be more valgus (turn inward) than men. If a person has wide hips, the ITB pain will usually be felt in the most lateral part of the leg (the center of the outer leg between the hip and knee). If not properly stretched, the ITB can become tight and shorten, which may cause pain above or below the knee joint, under the patella, or its entire length.

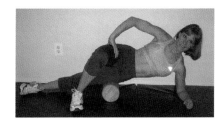

In addition to stretching, preventing ITB problems requires performing exercises that keep the hip musculature strong; such as side-lying leg abduction, hello dollies, or dirty dogs. While exercises to strengthen are important, maintaining flexibility is crucial. Specifically, stretch your quads (standing or lying), calves, hamstrings, glutes, and hips. I have found that using a foam roller directly on the ITB has proven to work quickly and effectively in restoring flexibility and rehabilitating the ITB, as well as alleviating knee pain.

If you are experiencing swelling, inflammation, or pain below your kneecap you may have sprained the patellar ligament: a condition known as **patella tendonitis**. Activities such as basketball, softball, volleyball, and soccer involve a lot of jumping and quick changes of direction. These activities place the patellar ligament under stress and may cause injury. Injury can also occur from overuse with activities such as running, sprinting, squatting, or speed walking. Patella tendonitis can occur if you fall and land heavily on your knees, as well. Always warm up for five minutes before exercise, include recovery time between workouts, perform balance exercises daily, wear supportive shoes, and avoid exercises or activities that cause pain. Wearing a supportive knee brace can provide your knee extra stability while recovering from a knee injury.

You do not have to be a football player to sustain an ACL injury. As a matter of fact, women (especially young girls) involved in sports such as soccer, basketball, skiing, and gymnastics are eight times more likely to sustain an ACL injury than men. During a woman's menstruation cycle, hormones are released that make her knee joint susceptible to injury. These hormones can cause a woman's joints to become looser and possibly unstable. It may be a good idea for women to avoid running, jumping, or heavy sports activities during this time.

An **ACL injury** occurs when the ligament is torn or excessively stretched by a sudden stop, a quick change of direction, a pivoting/twisting motion at the knee joint, or when there is a sudden impact to the front of the knee.

To ensure you are not included in the new ACL injury statistics, remember to keep your leg musculature strong and flexible. Wear supportive shoes, perform balance exercises daily, and add speed, agility, and quickness drills to your workout-especially if you play sports. If you have already sustained and ACL injury, wear a supportive brace to give your knee the stability it needs during exercise or while playing sports if you still feel any "giving way" symptoms.

<u>BACK PAIN</u>

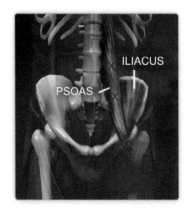

It is estimated that 80 percent of Americans suffer, at some point, from back pain each year. Most people choose painkillers and muscle relaxers to treat back pain symptoms after they occur, rather than use preventive measures such as correct posture, exercise and stretching regularly. You can

28

help prevent most back injuries by keeping your core and lower back muscles strong, your hip and leg muscles flexible, and maintaining good posture (not sitting in a slumped position) when sitting for long periods of time.

Two common, yet avoidable, problems I have found that cause back pain in executives are known as the **Psoas** and **Piriformis Syndromes**.

Back pain can occur when the iliopsoas muscle, which functions as a hip flexor, becomes tight and weak. As the muscle tightens, it shortens and pulls the hip joint down and forward in its socket, causing you to lose the natural curve in your lower back. Sitting for long periods of time; exercise programs emphasizing ab work, such as crunches, without including lower back exercises; sleeping in the side-lying fetal position; and a

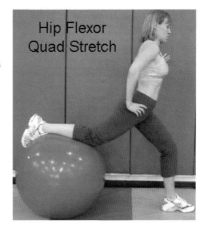

sedentary lifestyle can cause the iliopsoas to shorten and weaken. To prevent Psoas Syndrome, do hip flexor stretches and balance exercises to keep the muscle strong and flexible.

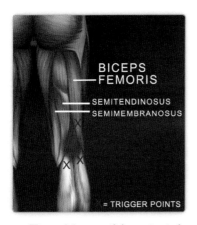

Back pain can also occur when hamstrings become weak and tight. This is especially true for men. When the hamstrings tighten they also shorten, pulling your butt and lower back toward the ground and flexing your hips forward. Thus, the natural curve in your lower back disappears. This makes it impossible for you to maintain good posture.

To address this, stretch your calf first, then perform the bicep femoris stretch, with an emphasis on proper form. Do these stretches daily, holding each for 30 seconds.

Next, make sure the piriformis is stretched and flexible. Talk about a pain in the butt! When the piriformis muscle becomes tight it aggravates the sciatic nerve, causing a painful condition known as Piriformis Syndrome or Sciatica.

This muscle is located deep in the hip/glute region in very close proximity to the sciatic nerve. When weak and tight, the piriformis muscle causes sciatic nerve pain. The pain originates in the lower back/buttocks and causes tingling, numbness, or shooting pain anywhere from the lower back all the way down the leg and into the big toe. A person who has long commutes to work, sits for long periods of time, travels, or runs for exercise without stretching is a prime candidate for this problem.

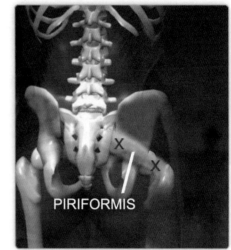

PIRIFORMIS

Test yourself by sitting at the edge of a chair and crossing one leg over the top of the knee on the opposite leg. If your hip feels stuck or in pain, if it is difficult to even cross one leg over the other, or if your knee is trying to point toward your head, you have a tight piriformis muscle. Stretches are crucial for preventing or alleviating this pain; so start by stretching your calf, hamstring, and piriformis muscles. Performing stretches of the bicep femoris, hip external rotator, low back, and IT Band will keep your back from tightening and losing its natural curve. When you perform the seated or lying piriformis stretch you relieve pressure and lengthen the sciatica nerve at the same time. Runners can restore and increase range of motion attaining a longer more fluid stride, as well.

Remember, muscle strength or length imbalance means that your muscles are playing "tug-of-war" with your body. Unless corrected with exercises and stretches, your muscles are literally fighting for control, and pulling your bones and joints out of alignment. When one muscle is weak and its opposing muscle is strong, or when one or more areas of the body become inflexible, some muscles become tight and weak while others stay long and flexible.

For example, a chiropractor can provide a temporary fix by adjusting your spine. However, if you don't stretch the muscles that pulled the spine out of alignment in the first place, these muscles will just pull the spine back out of alignment again. Like wise, if you don't strengthen the muscles that are weak,

Traci Trainer
T

your posture will suffer and predispose you to misalignment too. It is up to you to stretch and strengthen your muscles in order to maintain a healthy back. Performing body weight exercises such as superman crisscrosses, opposite arm/leg extensions, sky divers, prone scissors, floor bridges and back extensions will help keep your back strong. Proper posture while sitting and standing is also very important. When standing, pull your belly button back toward your spine. While sitting, do the same, but lean back in your chair at a 45 degree angle, if possible.

Spinal stenosis is a narrowing of the spinal canal resulting from aging, trauma, osteoarthritis, obesity, or heredity. If you are diagnosed with spinal stenosis, it is critical that you maintain the best posture possible at all times. Keeping core muscles strong will help you maintain proper posture, even when you are not thinking about it.

A **herniated disc** is one that protrudes out from between the vertebrae as a result of an acute injury (such as a car accident), improper form when lifting weights, or by months or years of uneven pressure on the disk caused by muscle imbalances. If you are diagnosed with a herniated disk, strengthen your core, maintain flexibility (especially in your legs and lower back), and use good posture at all times. Avoid exercises using heavy weights, which will put stress on your spine, as well as exercises in which you cannot maintain good form, such as the dead lift. Also, it is my recommendation that, you avoid seated back extension and seated abdominal crunch machines because they cause too much weighted sheer and compression force during back flexion and extension.

When you experience back pain, your first thought should be "I need to live pain-free," not "Shut up and deal with it." The combination of stretches that I have seen work for hundreds of clients, not only to relieve back pain, but, to keep the back muscles and spine healthy, follow this progression: calf, bicep femoris, piriformis, followed by low back. Also, many people find relief by performing one set of ten prone lying back extensions, holding for three seconds while in a "cobra-like" position.

You need to strengthen the muscles that support your back as well, by performing exercises such as the floor bridge, ball bridges, superman crisscross, opposite arm/leg extension, or the sky diver. In addition, maintain a strong core to help stabilize and support your lower back by adding prone scissors, properly performed crunches, toe reach crunches (elbows wide), leg and arm press, and or plank exercises. Remember, your abs, obliques, and glute muscles all support your lower back, so keep them strong. If your hamstrings, hip flexors, and piriformis get tight, they will compromise your posture and low back health. Keep them stretched!

Shoulder Pain

Shoulder problems have become all too common in this country. Men and women alike are suffering conditions such as rotator cuff tears, frozen shoulders, and bursitis. Remember, having surgery is not like getting new parts for your car. Sometimes our bodies form scar tissue after surgery which can lead to more surgery or, at the very least, a loss in our range of motion. It's not just baseball players, golfers, tennis players, weightlifters, or swimmers that suffer from shoulder problems. Included, are those of us approaching middle age. Imagine if you were unable to wash your hair, put on your bra, or get milk down from the top shelf of your fridge. Shoulder problems can severely limit your activities of daily living, and take anywhere from four months to a year to heal on average.

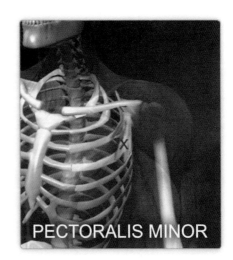
PECTORALIS MINOR

The supraspinatus, infraspinatus, subscapularis, and teres minor muscles are muscles of the rotator cuff. These muscles are responsible for correct shoulder joint mobility and rotating the shoulder. Impingement occurs when the rotator cuff or shoulder joint capsule (labrum) is pinched by part of the shoulder blade as the arm is lifted to the front, side, or behind your back. If your shoulder starts to hurt all of the

Traci Trainer

time, even when you aren't doing anything, you should see a doctor immediately. Ignoring the problem may lead to **frozen shoulder**, a condition where the joint capsule stiffens and causes you even more intense pain and misery. This creates a cyclical cycle of decreased range of motion and increased pain. The bursa that lies over the top of the rotator cuff can also become inflamed and cause pain with a rotator cuff tear or frozen shoulder. The pain is usually in the front of the shoulder or at the side of the arm around the deltoids (muscles on top of the shoulder) and can occur when lifting or reaching overhead. Depending on the severity of the problem, you may be treated with anti-inflammatory medication, sent to an occupational therapist, physical therapist, or even scheduled for surgery.

To prevent shoulder injuries, use the ball pec stretch daily. It will keep the muscles in the front of your shoulder flexible, reducing your risk of injury. Strengthen your upper body to give support to your shoulder by performing exercises elbow to elbow. By elbow to elbow, I mean exercise upper back muscles by performing rows, face pulls, and rear delt pulls, as well as triceps exercises, such as prone tricep extensions. Avoid tricep dips that put your shoulder in an unnatural position because you will be unable to maintain proper form. It is also my recommendation that you *never* perform overhead military presses. This exercise places the small stabilizing muscles of the shoulder in a position that is likely to cause impingement. If you are already experiencing

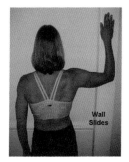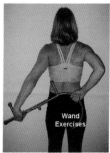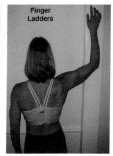 problems, perform wall slides, wand exercises, or finger ladder exercises to help with stiffness and to regain your lost range of motion. To strengthen your shoulder muscles, include internal and external rotation exercises with resistance or weight that you can tolerate while staying in a pain-free range of motion.

__NECK__

Stress and a slumped posture while sitting at a desk or in front of a computer all day can literally give you a pain in the neck. If you find yourself constantly rubbing the base of your neck where it connects to your shoulders or taking medications for headaches, you need to stretch the levator scapula muscle, upper trapezius, and scalene muscles that are tightening and pulling on your head and neck.

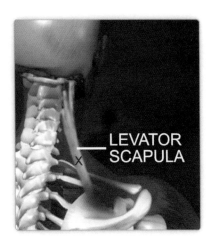

LEVATOR SCAPULA

Try leaning your head to one side while observing yourself in front of a mirror, forcing your right ear directly toward your right shoulder as far as you can,

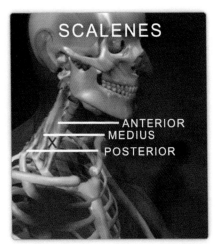

SCALENES

ANTERIOR
MEDIUS
POSTERIOR

without lifting your right shoulder to your ear. Repeat on the left side. Did one ear get closer to the shoulder than the other? If you answered yes, it is an indication that the muscles on one side of your neck are tighter than the muscles on the opposite side. Did your neck feel tight? If you answered yes, it is an indication that the above neck muscles are tight.

Now, I want you to retract your head by placing your first two fingers on your chin and pushing your head back, aligning it with your spine. Do you feel tightness, tenderness, or pain at the base of your skull where it attaches to your neck? Tenderness or pain there indicates that the cervical section of your spine is being affected by your poor posture habits. Imagine holding a bowling ball attached to the end of a stick and tilting that stick away from your body. The pain you imagine you would feel in your wrist is similar to the pain your neck feels when holding your head in a tilted position away from your body. Start doing chin retractions three times a day, 10 repetitions each time.

Ensure that the pillow you use when you sleep cradles your head, while providing adequate support for your neck. You can purchase a contour pillow or roll up a towel and place it inside your pillowcase at the base of your pillow. This will provide adequate support for your neck while it cradles your head.

Now, perform a chin retraction to put your head in line with your spine. Turn your head to the left and look directly down toward your nipple. Place your left hand on the top of your head and pull lightly. Repeat the process, looking to the right this time. Did you experience tightness or pain in you neck or upper shoulder blade region? If you answered yes, you need to stretch the levator scapula muscles. The levator muscle runs from the base of your skull to the top inner corner of your scapula (shoulder blade). Leaning your head forward for long periods of time causes the levator muscle to become overstretched, but tight where its tendon inserts under the shoulder blade.

A forward head and rounded shoulders indicate that your pec muscles are tight and your upper back/posterior shoulder muscles are too elongated, and therefore weak. Keep your neck healthy and pain-free by maintaining good posture, using chin retractions as needed, stretching the scalene and levator muscles, and providing extra support by strengthening the upper back and posterior shoulder muscles. Great exercises for the upper back and posterior shoulder include rows, face pulls, standing rear lateral raises, lat pullovers, lat pull downs, pulsed lateral raises, and serratus pulls.

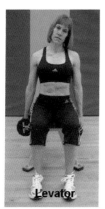
Levator

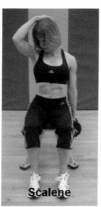
Scalene

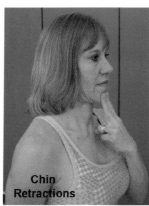
Chin Retractions

It's time to take inventory of your life's bumps, bruises, aches, and pains. Record them on the PAR-Q provided.

Chapter Four: Gumby is your new role model
Flexibility is your first key to success

Strength training is more important for women and flexibility training is more important for men. It is as if our brains weren't wired correctly for our physical needs. Most women hate strength training, but love to stretch. Men prefer strength training, and consider stretching a waste of time or a diversion from the main event. One trend I have noticed, for example, is that around age 15 boys' muscles begin to tighten, especially their hamstrings. And by age 35, men have sustained injuries and/or suffer from knee or back pain. The back pain can usually be attributed to overly tight hamstrings; while knee pain, plantar fasciitis, and heel pain can usually be attributed to overly tight calf muscles.

I want you to picture a muscle stretching from one bone to the next crossing a joint. If the muscle becomes either tight or weak, it will cause a muscle imbalance around the joint. This increases the injury probability at one of the joints – that is, unless the muscle itself decides to tear. The joint with the least muscular support is usually the one injured. For example, if you have an overly tight calf muscle, an injury will probably occur either to the ankle, knee or both. Say you have developed strong supporting muscles surrounding the knee, then it is your foot/ankle complex that will more likely suffer an injury.

Now I want you to picture pulling on the ends of a rubber band. Watch it stretch and then return to its original shape. Tie a few knots in the rubber band and then try pulling on the ends. You will notice that the knots continue to tighten while the areas closest to the knots weaken. Eventually, the rubber band will break next to a knot where the section can no longer take the pressure. Your muscles act in a similar manner. If you keep the muscles stretched they will not develop knots and render themselves useless to perform their necessary function and become prone to injury. Instead, the muscle will stretch at both ends and return to its original shape. If you continue to boast that you don't need to stretch, at least research and find a good physical therapist in your area. Thus, it is not a matter of if, but when an injury will occur. When you don't stretch, more knots continue to form in the muscle, getting tighter with each use. The muscle will eventually tear or cause a joint injury. For a while you may continue to run, jump, play tennis and otherwise function normally. But one day, the muscle that is too tight will let you know that it has had enough of your mistreatment. If you think you are too busy now to make time for stretching, consider working a two-hour physical therapy appointment three times a week into your schedule.

Now close your eyes and think thoughts of taffy or silly putty. I have selected five primary stretches, placing them in a particular order for your beginning stretching routine. I have based my selection on the successes I have witnessed with hundreds of executives. These successes have ranged from better stride length while running, to completely alleviating knee pain. It is my hope that by using this same routine, you too will have similar success, or better yet, prevent an injury from happening in the first place. The calf, bicep femoris, and piriformis stretches can all be performed in your office. If you are unable to make time for a workout during the day, at least devote three minutes to stretch these muscles.

After two weeks of stretching daily (including Sunday), you will start to feel some of the sharpness dissipate when performing these stretches. After four weeks, the muscle should become more flexible and easier to stretch. You may need to continue stretching some muscles longer than four weeks before you feel success if those muscles were already in bad shape. It is easier to maintain strength and flexibility than it is to regain it.

It is very important that you breathe and relax during each stretch. Not only can too much pressure build up behind your eyes, it can rob your muscle of the one thing it needs; oxygenated blood. In a 2006 study conducted by the Institute of Specialized Ophthalmology, it was discovered that holding your breath during exercises can increase your risk of developing glaucoma. It was discovered that pressure behind the eye can rise as high as 90 percent during certain exercises.

Your feet take heavy pounding throughout a normal day. With that said, it is not surprising that my clients have found more immediate success starting with calf stretches and working their way up rather than with neck stretches working their way down. Unfortunately, most people do calf stretches with bad form.

Usually the person lifts the heel off the ground, or the person moves in and out of the stretch before allowing enough time for the stretch to occur. I start everyone off with a calf stretch by placing the foot in a dorsiflexed position, limiting the chances that the stretch will be performed with bad form. You can do this stretch using a curb outside, a step, a wall, a Prostretch®, or any elevated surface that allows you to put your foot in a dorsiflexed position.

After placing the foot to be stretched, walk your other foot forward. Stand with good posture and lean over without your butt sticking out. If the stretch is too strong, simply back off and reposition your foot with less elevation. If you need more of a stretch, walk the foot you are not stretching forward, passing the foot you are stretching. If you discover that your toes point away from your body when performing your squat assessment or you notice that you stand, walk, or run like a duck, it is an indication that the peroneal muscles are tight and in need of stretching. The peroneal is part of the calf complex but is not in the back of your leg; it runs parallel on the outside of your shin. When tight, the muscle pulls your toes away from the midline of your body and doesn't allow proper dorsiflexion to occur. To stretch this muscle, point your toes slightly inward toward the midline of your body and walk forward; hold for 30 seconds.

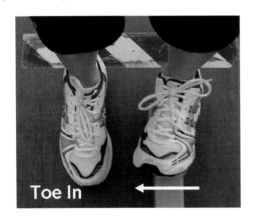
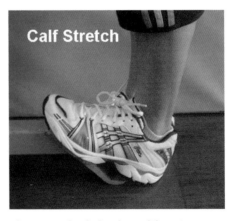

The stretch selected next is the bicep femoris stretch. It is the ultimate hamstring stretch. It's unlike anything you have ever felt before, but it works! Prepare for some discomfort, but keep in mind that this stretch may save you from back pain or alleviate current back pain. When stretching the hamstring is uncomfortable, most people cheat by changing the position of their hips or feet to make the stretch more comfortable. It is best to use proper form and move carefully and slowly into the stretch. Stop at the first sign of discomfort, then hold your position until the muscle starts to feel like it is relaxing.

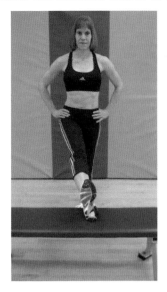
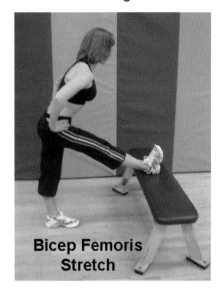

Bicep Femoris Stretch

It is important that the foot remaining on the ground stays straight so ensure your toes point straight ahead at all times. Do not elevate your other leg to hip height or the stretch will be ineffective. Use a bench, chair, step, or curb instead. Move the elevated leg until it is midline to your body, then using your leg muscles – not your hands – pull your toes back toward your face. This is usually where you notice the first sign of discomfort and for some, the calf still feels tight even though it was stretched first. Now breathe! Most people stop breathing at the first sign of discomfort; and begin to make pained facial expressions. Relax your face and concentrate on breathing. When you breathe, oxygenated blood flows to the muscle and helps it to stretch. Do not be alarmed if you feel this stretch in your calf or behind your knee at first. As your calf becomes more flexible this stretch will move from the calf, to behind the knee, and eventually reach your hamstring. It will continue to move as far as your butt. Keeping your back flat and your belly button pulled back toward your spine, hinge at the hip and lean forward until the first sign of discomfort is felt. Do not round your back. You may not be able to lean forward if you were unable to get past the discomfort when you initially pulled your toes back toward your face. If a mirror is available, perform this stretch where you can view yourself from the side. If your tail is tucking under like a scared dog and your body is forming the shape of the letter "C," do your body a favor and do this stretch daily until you regain an upright proper posture.

As an executive, you spend a lot of time sitting. Therefore, the seated piriformis is your next stretch. Sit forward on the edge of your chair or bench, place your feet hip-width apart, and point your toes straight ahead. Cross one foot over the top of the knee of the opposite leg. Using one hand, lightly press down on the medial knee of the elevated leg. Using the other hand, pull up on the heel of the elevated leg. Hold this position for approximately 10 seconds. You may notice a catch in your outer hip, tightness on the inside of your thigh, or a stretch occurring in your butt. Release your hands and reposition them by grabbing your shin. Pull your belly button back toward your spine and keep your back straight. Lean forward, hinging at the hips, until you feel discomfort coming from a small area in your butt. For some it feels as if being stabbed with an ice pick, and for others it feels like a dull ache; for those of us who stretch frequently, it just feels good. You are now stretching the muscles surrounding your sciatic nerve. If you are making ugly faces and holding your breath, please relax your face and breathe.

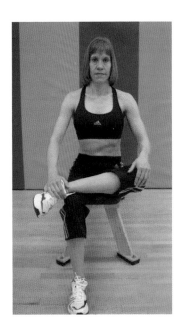
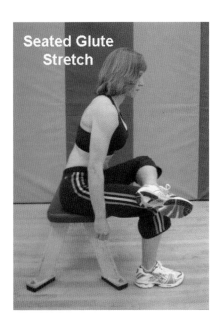

Seated Glute Stretch

I recommend that your fourth choice be the low back stretch. Lie on your back and extend your arms to each side to form the letter "T". Pull your belly button back toward your spine. Use your abdomen muscles to lift your legs into a bent-knee position with your feet off the floor. Keep your knees together and use

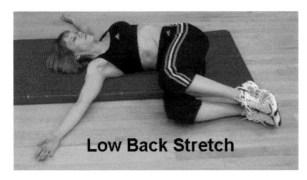

Low Back Stretch

your abdomen muscles to slowly lower your legs off to one side until they reach the floor. If your opposite arm lifts off the floor as you lower your knees, this is an indication that your low back and pec muscles are tight. For now, place your hand on

that hip to avoid damage to the front of the shoulder or pec muscles, and make sure that you add the ball-pec stretch to your stretching routine. Hold this stretch for 30 seconds. Use your abdomen muscles to pull your legs back to their elongated starting point. Repeat the stretch by lowering your legs to the opposite side. This will ensure that your spine is in proper alignment for the next stretch. Avoid moving your legs from side to side, as if you were a windshield wiper.

To protect your rotator cuff, stretch your pec and anterior shoulder muscles by using the ball-pec stretch (you can also use a chair, couch, or bench). Get down on your hands and knees. Keep your belly button pulled back toward your spine

and your head in line with your spine (do not drop your head). Raise one arm straight out to the side bent at 90 degrees, and rest your elbow on top of the stability ball. Lightly push your shoulder down toward the floor, while turning your head away from the ball. Although some experience sharp pain in the front of the shoulder, this is meant to

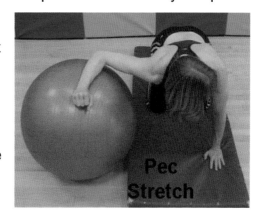

Pec Stretch

be a nice, gentle stretch that will slowly spread throughout the pec muscle over the next 30 seconds.

In order to select the remaining stretches, you will need to refer to the information that you documented on your PAR-Q. Keep in mind that these stretches will be selected using your current personal posture assessment, which indicates which of your muscles are now overly tight. Go easy on yourself at first with the understanding that, as time passes, the stretch will feel less painful/sharp and your range of motion will increase.

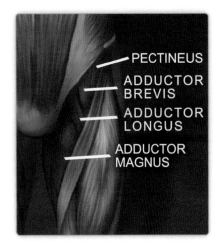

If your PAR-Q indicates that you rounded your back and tucked your butt under like a dog in trouble, then the back and inside of your legs are tight. The bicep femoris stretch has already been selected for you, so you must add the adductor on a ball stretch to stretch the inside of your thighs. Tight adductors are very common in women, but can become tight on men as well, and possibly cause a groin pull – ouch! Sit on a stability ball and place your feet hip-width apart and point your toes straight ahead. Pull your belly button back toward your spine for stability. Extend one leg out to the side while keeping your other foot flat on the floor, toes pointed straight ahead. Lock your knee. You may feel the stretch at this point. If not, roll slowly forward on the ball while maintaining good posture. Do not lean your body away from the extended leg. As soon as you feel the stretch, hold for 30 seconds. Roll the ball back to its original position, bend your knee and pull your extended leg back to the original starting position. Now stretch the adductors of the opposite leg. You will also need to add the adductor stretch to your routine if, on your

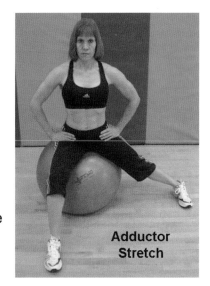

Adductor Stretch

Par-Q, you indicated that your knees tried to touch each other during the squat assessment. This would also indicate that the muscles on the insides of your thighs (adductor complex) are tight.

If your PAR-Q indicates that you arched your back and stuck your butt out during the squat, then your hip flexor muscles and your back muscles that attach and run parallel to your spine are tight. This is probably caused by sitting for long periods of time, or not stretching properly after you run or exercise. If this is the case, you will need to add the hip flexor and erector spinae stretches to your routine.

When performing the hip flexor stretch, keep one foot on the floor and elevate the other foot onto a bench or chair. Looking straight ahead, pull your belly button back toward your spine, then lean until the stretch is felt in the crease of your upper front thigh. After holding for 30 seconds, repeat the stretch on the opposite leg.

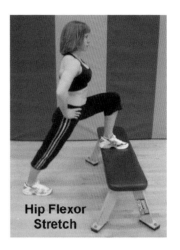

Hip Flexor Stretch

The erector spinae stretch is difficult for some people to perform, so I am including an alternative stretch. Sit on the floor with your right leg extended. Pull your belly button back toward your spine. Bend your left knee and place your left foot on the outside of your right knee. Bend your right elbow and place it on the outside of your elbow against the outside of the raised left knee. Push your right elbow against your left knee. Twist your trunk to the left until the stretch is felt and then hold the position for 30 seconds. Repeat the stretch on the opposite side. If you were unable to get into proper form with this stretch, then try this next option. Lie on your back. Bring your knees to your chest and hug your knees with your arms. Pull your knees down toward your chest, then toward your head. Hold for 30 seconds.

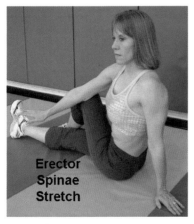

Erector Spinae Stretch

If your PAR-Q indicates that your hips shifted to one side during your squat, then your adductors on the same side as the shift and your piriformis and IT Band on the opposite side of the shift are tight. The piriformis stretch has already been selected for you. Add to your routine, a stretch for your adductor on the same side as your hip shifts.

If your PAR-Q indicates that your hands fell forward and you struggled to keep your arms in line with your ears when you performed the squat, then your chest muscles are tight. If your toes pointed away from your body (externally rotated) or your heels rose off the floor, it indicates that your calves are tight. If your knees bowed outward, your bicep femoris and piriformis are tight. These are common problems that have been addressed in the first five stretches selected for you.

Injuries go hand in hand with sports. If you are a weekend warrior, perform specific stretches for your sport of choice to reduce your risk of injury and improve your performance. If you participate in any of the following sports, add these stretches to your routine if they are not already included:

Running: calf/bicep femoris/piriformis/lying glute/IT band

Soccer: calf/bicep femoris/lying quad/hip flexor/adductor

Golf: side stretches/erector spinae/IT band/triceps/forearm/pec

Tennis: calf/bicep femoris/adductor/pec

Softball: calf/bicep femoris/lying quad/low back

Swimming: calf/pec/lat

Basketball: calf/bicep femoris/lying quad/IT band/pec

The difference between a weekend warrior who participates in a sport for fun and recreation, and an athlete who plays professionally, is that an athlete properly trains for his/her sport. If you remain unconvinced that the above stretches are necessary when participating in a recreation sport, just take a look at the common injuries associated with each sport:

Running: runner's knee, ITB Syndrome, shin splints, stress fractures, pulled or torn hamstrings, sprained ankles, plantar fasciitis, Achilles tendonitis

Soccer: ankle sprains, Achilles tendonitis, pulled groin, pulled or torn hamstrings, ITB Syndrome, ACL tear or meniscal tears

Tennis: back and knee pain, rotator cuff tears, tennis elbow, ankle sprains, calf and Achilles tendon injuries

Softball: ACL or meniscal tears, ankle sprains, rotator cuff and knee tendonitis

Swimming: back, knee, and hip pain, shoulder tendonitis, vertebral fractures

Basketball: patella tendonitis, Achilles tendonitis, ankle sprains, ACL or meniscus tears, numerous shoulder injuries

I've saved golf for last, because the injury list is long and the sport is common among executives. The golf swing is a complex move that requires many muscles to execute. It uses 22 muscles for the forward motion of the swing alone! All core muscles, hamstrings, quads, upper back, shoulder, forearm, as well as all of the muscles in the wrists and fingers, are required to execute a golf swing. If any muscle is tight, it will affect the precision of the golf swing and place the golfer at a higher risk of injury. Golf-related injuries include back pain, herniated discs, elbow tendonitis or bursitis, torn rotator cuffs, rotator cuff tendonitis, shoulder bursitis or impingement, torn meniscus, arthritis of the knee, patellar pain, and carpal tunnel syndrome.

Provided on the next page are additional stretches that you may choose to incorporate into your stretching routine after you experience the benefits from your initial stretch routine.

Pec Stretch

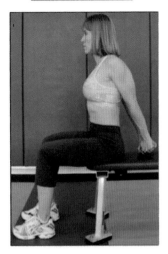

Mid Back Stretch

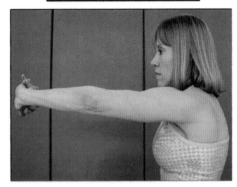

Lying Glute Stretch

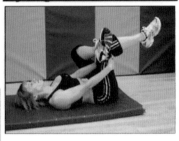

Remember:
*relax shoulders
*pull leg back toward chest using bicep

Tricep Stretch   ## Lat

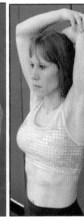 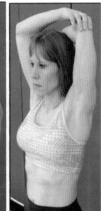

Lying Quad stretch

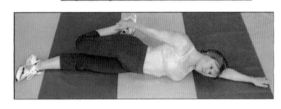

Bicep Stretch

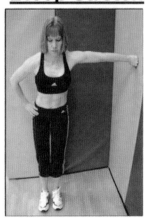

Forearm stretch

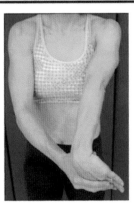

Remember to relax and breathe during all stretches!

IT Band stretch

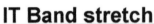
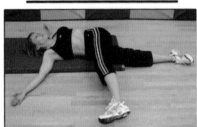

46

Traci Trainer

Chapter Five: Breathe!

Building Cardio Endurance

I currently lecture and train for the Executive Learning Office of the U.S. Navy. I have developed an executive health program to meet the needs of their senior active-duty officers, as well as senior executive civilian personnel, ranging in age from 35 to 70, in all branches of service. During my strength training basics lecture, I present a slide that tells them simply to *breathe*. It never fails to create a room full of laughter. In the back of my mind I am thinking, "Just wait until tonight," because my first training session is always the 10 minute routine which I developed to train people to breathe, build their cardio endurance, and at the same time take and inch or two off their waist. It sounds easy enough. How difficult can breathing and 10 minutes of exercise be? Well, you will have the opportunity to find that out for yourself. All you need is a stopwatch and a jump rope. The routine is broken down into 10 one-minute intervals. You can do just about anything for one minute, right?

When a person sits for long periods of time they tend to develop what I call shallow or neck breathing. This type of breathing allows only a small amount of oxygen into the lungs. What are you doing right now? You are probably sitting with your belly protruding (Pull your belly button back toward your spine – every second counts!) and your chest barely rising and falling with each breath. Breathing this way day in and day out doesn't exercise the diaphragm and prepare the lungs to be able to do their job when it comes time to exert energy. If you are saying to yourself, "Yeah, but I can run for three miles just fine," you are what I call a hamster in a wheel. If your current cardio routine involves only walking, running, or using the same machine each time you exercise, you are becoming a pattern breather because your body never has demands placed on it. If your body could speak, it would say, "Here we go again. No need to stress out. He/she's just going to read a magazine while on the elliptical for a half hour." This is exactly the reason people plateau and then become exceedingly frustrated when they are unable to achieve their goals, even though they exercise daily. Changes will occur in your body as it adapts to the new demands forced upon it; you must constantly change your cardio routine in order to build and maintain cardio endurance.

You will notice when performing the 10 minute routine for the first time that you will become short of breath around minute three. Knowing this information will not help. Only building cardio endurance by breathing properly during exercise will.

Jumping rope may or may not come easy to you at first, but it has been my experience that the third time is the charm. It should only take performing the routine three times a week for four weeks to become comfortable with it and get results. Remember to take a 24 hour break in between. It doesn't matter what style of rope you choose, only that the length is correct. When you stand in the center of the rope, the handles should come up to your armpits. Please note, when you jump rope, it should not appear to those around you that you are trying to develop hurdler skills. Your elbows should stay close to your sides as you use your wrist to flick the rope. Only jump high enough to pass the rope under your feet. Breathe in through your nose for three counts and exhale through your mouth for three counts. Most people find it easy to breathe in, but difficult to control their exhale. You may experience dizziness the first few times you do your routine, because you're not used to taking in a lot of oxygen. This is exactly why you need to build cardio endurance. So don't give up! It would be a good idea to take in deep breaths throughout the day, whenever you think about it.

I implore you to keep your belly button pulled back toward your spine at all times. You may find this especially hard to do during jumping jacks. Every time your belly pushes out, please pull it back in. It is your abdomen muscles job to protect your lumbar spine and keep your organs from being juggled around in your belly like balls in a lotto machine. It is also important when performing "ice skaters" that you keep your feet together. When performing "ski jumps," your toes should stay pointed straight ahead when landing to protect your knees.

Although your body may feel as if it has been run over by a truck, it still has a little energy reserved. To prove it, you will end this torture with three plyometric jumps, performing 10 reps each. Landing mechanics are crucial when performing plyometric exercises. Always start with your feet hip-width apart and your toes pointed straight ahead. Then explode with all of the energy you can muster. Make sure you land on your toes from your original starting position, with your leg muscles contracted.

Completing four weeks of the 10 minute routine is a good start. But like all good things, it must come to an end. Continue to change your cardio routine in order to maintain the endurance you have built, while continuing to make gains. Alternate your choices on cardio training days. For example, run on Monday, use the elliptical on Wednesday, and bicycle on Friday. After seeing my personal results, as well as my clients' results, I have become a strong supporter of interval training. Interval training during cardio exercises means varying the levels of intensity during a workout period. Now it is time to get creative. When you're on the elliptical, go forward, backward, use the handles or don't hold on at all. Instead, learn to balance yourself while in motion. When using the treadmill, go forward, backward, side step, use the incline, or alternate speeds. Use a bike for a few minutes, switch to the elliptical, and finish with the treadmill. Run for a distance, walk and sprint, side-step, run backwards, skip, or do carioca steps, then run again. Get on the treadmill or elliptical for a few minutes, then jump rope for a few minutes, alternating between the two. Think outside the box and you will find that the possibilities are endless. Over time, the body will adapt to whatever you challenge it to do. Interval training will change your body from the inside out. You will look better, feel better, and improve your body's overall health, all at the same time.

10 Minute Cardio Routine

Perform 1 minute of each exercise:
Single jumps with rope
Running jumps with rope
Jumping Jacks
Ice Skaters:
(side to side jumps feet together)
Single jumps with rope
Running jumps with rope
Jumping Jacks
Ski jumps:
(lateral jump into single leg balance)
Single jumps with rope
10 reps Squat Jumps
10 reps Butt Kicks
10 reps Tuck Jumps

Squat Jumps

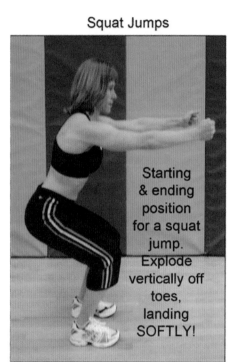

Starting & ending position for a squat jump.
Explode vertically off toes, landing SOFTLY!

Butt Kicks

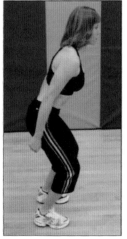 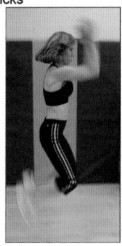

Tuck Jumps

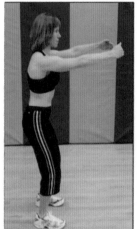 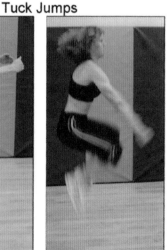

Chapter Six: No Excuses!

Can't resist resistance training

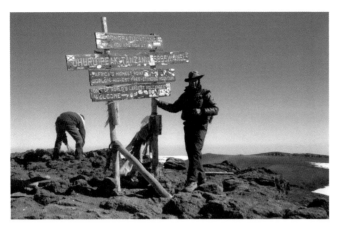

If you are in good shape when you hit 60, you will probably be able to out-perform most of todays' 20-year-olds, as long as your bones and joints hold out. Some of my 60 plus-year-old clients are still bicycling, rollerblading, and boogie boarding. One client, a 63-year-old senior executive, decided he wanted to climb Kilimanjaro. I did not discourage him because I knew he was in the best shape of his life. I enjoyed the photo he sent of himself, standing proudly at the summit – but I enjoyed even more his e-mail that read, "I am a successful climber/summitter of the big mountain in Africa, Kilimanjaro! In fact, I was in better shape for this kind of activity than all 26 people … rivaled only by a 25-year-old."

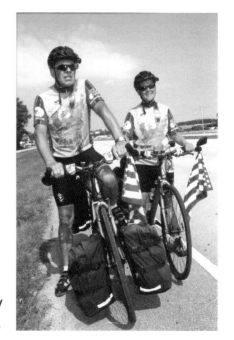

Sometimes I am asked, "Where do you get your energy?" I always smile and tell this story. My mom and stepfather came for a visit when I lived in Cherry Point, N.C. My driveway became the jumping off spot for the greatest ride of their lives. Although they were in their late 50's, they bicycled 9,749 miles across the United States and back again. They averaged 60 miles per day and carried all the gear they would need in order to camp out if they ever had to stop unexpectedly for the night. They bicycled into my driveway seven months later, followed by television camera crews and newspaper reporters. My mother, now 20 pounds lighter, said to the press, "I feel more like 38 than 58." I hope by sharing these examples I have inspired you, and shown that your age shouldn't hold you back. It is only poor physical condition that can, and will.

In each of the cases above, strength training played a major role and should be included in every exercise program. However, doing "any ol' exercise any ol' way" can do more harm than good; don't let your ego dictate your exercise program and just start throwing some weight around. Instead, use the following guidelines to ensure your resistance-training program is a success:

- 5 to10 minute warm-ups are essential
- Check all five body positions before you perform any
   exercise:

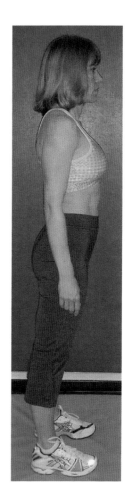

   1. feet hip-width apart and toes pointed straight ahead
   2. knees slightly flexed (never locked out)
   3. hips in neutral position
   4. shoulders retracted and depressed
   5. head in line with your spine
- Always keep your belly button pulled back toward your spine
- Never sacrifice form to add more weight
- Change your exercise program every four to five weeks
- Once you have mastered an exercise, it is time to progress
- Start with low weight and high reps when performing a new
   exercise
- Make sure that all body movements are slow and controlled
- Always work opposing muscle groups
- Challenge your body by changing position and type of
   resistance
- Make it proprioceptively challenging (force your body to
   maintain balance)
- Choose at least one exercise for each core muscle group

Although the focus is not on cardio, it is still necessary to get your heart rate up on resistance-training days. Your body needs a good five to 10 minutes warm-up to circulate oxygenated blood throughout the body and elevate your heart rate. I'm a huge fan of making the most of your warm-up, and have given you the 10 minute routine as an example of a dynamic warm-up. Use your warm-up as an opportunity to maximize caloric burn. In other words, don't just walk around the block, power walk around the block. Utilize the interval-training techniques you learned in chapter five to create a varied, as well as effective, warm-up routine. You can also use interval training during your entire workout by alternating resistance exercises with small bouts of cardio exercises.

Interval Training Example Routine

Jump Rope for 60-seconds

Split Squat Jumps: Start in a lunge position (ensure your forward knee is not over your toes and your shoulders are in line with your hips). Explode into a jump. Switch foot position mid-air, landing into a lunge. Perform **15 reps**.

Russian Twist: Sit on the floor or a bench with your knees together in a bent knee position and your toes pointing toward the ceiling. Lean back until you feel your abs engage. Hold the weight shoulder height in front of you with your elbows slightly bent. Keeping your shoulders squared, twist to your right. Use your abs to pull the weight back to the center (readjust your shoulders if necessary) before twisting to the left. Perform **15 reps.**

V-sits: Sit on a bench while balancing on your butt. Assume a bent knee position with your feet elevated and your toes pulled back toward your face. Keeping your shoulders retracted and depressed and your head in line with your spine, move your legs down and up. Perform **25 reps.**

Squat Thrusts: Stand with your feet hip width apart and toes pointed straight ahead. Explode into a squat jump and drop immediately into a pushup position. Jump into a deep squat, ensuring that your knees remain inside your arms. Quickly explode into your next repetition. Perform **15 reps.**

Toe Reach Crunches: Lie on your back with both legs straight in the air. Point your toes back toward your face. Pointing your fingers toward your toes, pulse upward into a crunch (attempt to reach past your toes). Perform **20 reps.**

Seated Hammer Curls: While you are either seated or standing, hold a dumbbell in each hand by your side, elbows slightly bent. Raise the dumbbells up and over your shoulder as if raising a hammer. Stop when the dumbbells are next to your ears. Return the dumbbells to their original position as slowly as possible without swinging your arms. Perform **15 reps**.

Prone Scissors: Lie face down on the floor with your arms crossed under your face and your forehead resting on your arms. Raise your legs until your thighs are off the floor. Point your toes toward the floor then open and close your legs as if they were a pair of scissors. Perform **25 reps.**

Squat Flings for 60 seconds.

Rear Delt Pulls: Sit on a bench. Hold a resistance tube with both arms directly in front of you, elbows slightly bent. Keep your shoulders retracted and depressed (do not elevate your shoulders) and pull the tube out and back toward your chest while squeezing your shoulder blades together. Return your arms to their original position. Perform **15 reps.**

When You're Up Pushups: Assume the pushup position then push up and hold. Lower yourself to the floor. This time push up only half way and hold. Continue to push all the way up and then lower all the way back down. Control your speed by repeating this rhyme during each repetition: "When you're up you're up and when you're down you're down; but when you're only half way up you're neither up nor down." Perform **8-10 reps.**

Prone Dumbbell Tricep Extensions: Lie face down on a bench, keeping your head in line with your spine. Holding a dumbbell in each hand, raise your elbows and keep them tight to your sides. Kick both dumbbells back at the same time, stopping when they are in line with your body. Return the dumbbells slowly to their original position ensuring you only move from elbow to wrist. Perform **15 reps**.

Lateral jumps for 60 seconds

Squat to Front Raise: Using a weighted bar or dumbbells, lower yourself into a squat position while raising your arms into a front raise. If you are using a bar, your palms will be facing the floor. If you are using dumbbells, your palms will be facing each other. Remember to keep your elbows slightly flexed as you raise the weight in front of you. Perform **15 reps**.

Single Leg Calf Raises: Stand on your right foot while holding onto a ball or stable surface (ensure the foot on the ground is straight). Wrap your left foot behind your right ankle. Lift and lower your heel while making sure your foot stays pointed straight ahead and does not externally rotate. Repeat using your left foot. Perform **15 reps on each leg.**

Clap Jacks for 60 seconds

Repeat circuit then stretch: calf/hamstring/quad/lying glute/low back and pec.

Keep in mind that not all exercises are good for you. The exercises listed below are riskier than others. Either the mechanics of the exercises are dangerous to your frame if not performed correctly, or the exercises are easily replaced by other exercises that get better results with less risk of injury.

Sit-ups: Sit-ups account for 63 percent of all weight-lifting related emergency room visits. Locking your hands behind your head and pulling on your neck can torque your cervical vertebrae and cause neck pain. Crossing your hands in front of your chest and doing sit-ups will bow your mid-back and can cause you to lose the natural curve in your lower back. Then as your hip flexors tighten, lower back pain may result. Sit-ups are also one of the least-effective ab exercises. Bicycles will work your abs and obliques 250% more efficiently. If you want a challenge, do bicycles on a BOSU® balance trainer.

Behind-the-neck lat pull-downs & military overhead presses: Avoid any behind-the-neck exercises. They can stress your cervical discs and vertebrae, causing neck pain. These two exercises also rotate the shoulders into a position that impinges and strains the rotator cuff muscles. Instead, perform lat pull-downs by pulling the bar to your chest. It is safer and gives you a greater range of motion. One of the most poorly performed exercises is the military overhead press. First, it puts the small stabilizing muscles of the rotator cuff between a rock and a hard place. Literally! Imagine sliding a string back and forth over the edge of a table. Eventually the string will break. When your arms extend past the shoulders to lift the weights overhead, the rotator cuff gets pinched between the clavicle and the humerus. Poor form may precipitate lower back injury, as well. In addition, when the weights are lifted overhead, the lifter usually forgets to keep his abs tight, locks his knees, and pushes his butt out. This can cause back hyperextension, which can lead to disk herniation in the lumbar spine. To work the shoulders and reduce the risk of injury, hands should be turned so that the palms are facing each other.

Straight bar curls: This exercise locks your arms into an unnatural, palm-up position which puts stress on your elbow joints and can lead to elbow tendinitis. Perform bicep curls using free weights. Start with your palms facing inward and twist into a curl on the way up to the shoulder. Never lock out your elbows when performing any exercise. Always keeping the elbows slightly flexed will reduce the risk of developing tendinitis.

Seated pec decks: At the physical therapy clinic where I worked, I was often shown workout programs that had been developed by personal trainers for their female clients. Each and every one of those women who had pec decks or pec flys in their program ended up having rotator-cuff surgery. And men are not exempt from this problem. These exercises put the shoulder in an unstable position, placing excessive stress on the anterior shoulder joint and its connective tissue. Replace these exercises with pushups. Pushups reduce the risk of injury by using your body weight to strengthen your chest. I would also recommend replacing the bench press with the incline press, using lighter weight and more repetition.

Smith machine squats: The alignment of this machine causes unnatural arched movements throughout your body frame, and puts stress on your knees, shoulders, and lower back. Replace Smith machine squats with body-weight squats.

When you routinely exercise with proper form, your body will stay in the five body positions from your first repetition to your last. **Never** sacrifice form for added weight! Before you add weight, see if you are able to do the same exercise using only one arm, one leg, or while standing/sitting on an unstable surface such as a BOSU® balance trainer or a stability ball. If you are successful, it proves you have mastered the current weight and can safely add additional weight. Don't go crazy when increasing weight! Add small increments to avoid injury. When you want to increase weight in exercises that use your body weight, simply reduce the number of points of contact. For example, a plank is a body-weight exercise where all four limbs are in contact with the floor. To add weight to the plank, lift an arm, a leg, or one of each off the floor. With that said, you would definitely not want to perform a plank for the first time by lifting one arm and the opposite leg off the floor. First, master a simple plank with all limbs in contact with the floor, and then advance to the next level plank. Eventually, you will advance to the most difficult level plank. This technique is called the "crawl, walk, run" progression.

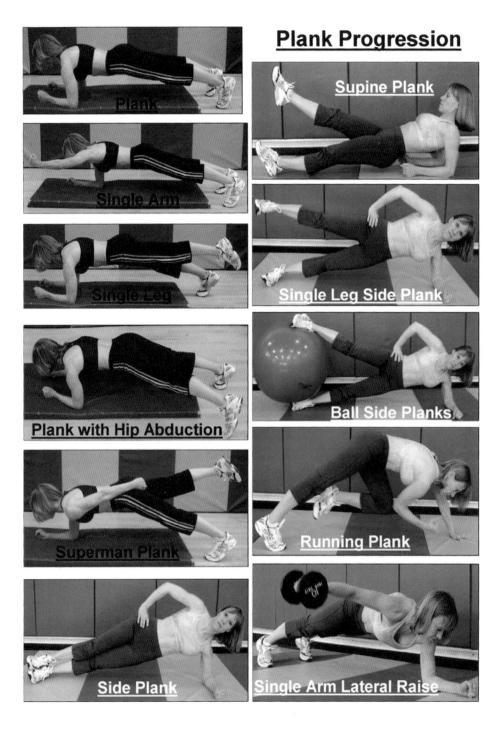

Plank Progression

Plank

Single Arm

Single Leg

Plank with Hip Abduction

Superman Plank

Side Plank

Supine Plank

Single Leg Side Plank

Ball Side Planks

Running Plank

Single Arm Lateral Raise

Dip Progression

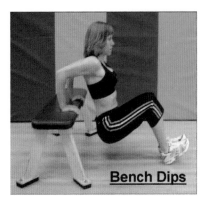

Bench Dips

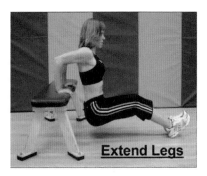

Extend Legs

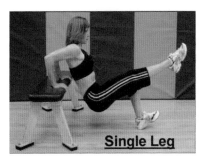

Single Leg

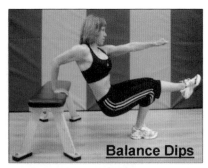

Balance Dips

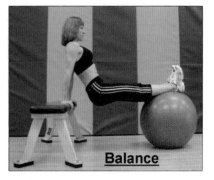

Balance

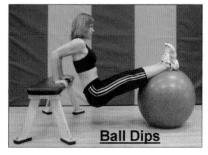

Ball Dips

Remember:
*keep abs drawn in
*dip down until arms form a right angle
*set shoulders back and down
*never dip past a right angle

Traci Trainer

Progressing exercises at the correct time is very important. You want to avoid injury and frustration but, at the same time, you won't get results you want and may plateau if you don't challenge yourself. It will take approximately four weeks for you to master the exercises in your program. You can progress naturally and avoid a plateau by changing your workout routine every four to five weeks. If you have been performing a basic bench dip with your knees at a 90 degree angle for four weeks and the exercise has become easy, simply extend your legs to increase the amount of weight your triceps are lifting. It will feel like a whole new exercise. Just remember to progress slowly. Staying challenged, without frustration or injury, is key.

When starting a new exercise, use a light weight and perform two sets of fifteen reps. Your primary focus should be on using correct form. After you have completed the movement correctly 30 times, your brain and nervous system will have gotten the message then you can perform this movement safely. Using light weight with high reps gives your brain time to warm up the nervous system and recruit all muscles necessary to perform the movement safely. Using heavy weight does not give the brain and nervous system enough time to learn the correct movement. One or more muscles may not fire at the correct time, increasing your risk of injury. For maximum caloric burn, all movement should be slow and controlled and rest periods between 0-30 seconds.

When designing your exercise routine remember you must always work opposing muscle groups to avoid muscle imbalances and injury. For example, if you work your biceps you should also work your triceps. Muscles work together. In this case, when the bicep contracts its reciprocal muscle, the tricep, must lengthen and vice versa. These two muscles will become imbalanced if you only strengthen the bicep, and leave the tricep weak and unable to support the elbow joint as needed. One of the most common muscle imbalances occurs when a person performs only abdominal exercises and ignores the lower back completely. This can result in injury and pain anywhere from your neck to your lower back. A total body resistance-training program will ensure that you will work all of your major muscle groups and keep your body in better balance.

A total body resistance-training template is provided for you on the next page. Use this training notes page to formulate and annotate your own specific warm-ups, stretches and exercises.

Training Notes

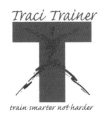

Warm-Up
5-10 minute warm-up

Cardio
Do your choice of cardio on non-resistance training days

STRETCH EVERY DAY 1 Set with 30 second hold (for each of the below stretches)	

CORE	Exercise	Sets	Reps	Weight
Lower Back				
Hips/Glute				
Abs				
Oblique				
Balance				

Strength	Exercise	Sets	Reps	Weight
Chest				
Upper/Middle Back				
Shoulders				
Biceps				
Triceps				
Legs				

Notes: 1. Don't forget your 24 hour recovery period between workouts.
2. All movement should be slow and controlled.
3. Keep rest periods between 0-30 seconds

Remember to challenge your body by changing your body position or the type of resistance you are using. You can choose to stand, sit, lie prone, lie supine, kneel, or even stagger your stance.

If you become bored with weight machines try free weights, resistance tubes, weighted bars, ankle weights, or medicine balls.

Change body position, type of resistance,
or make it proprioceptively challenging!

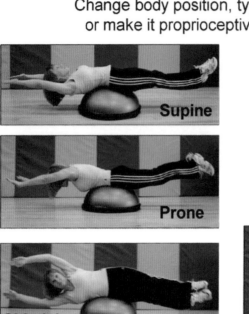

Supine

Prone

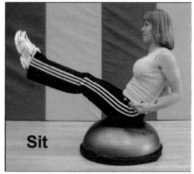

Sit

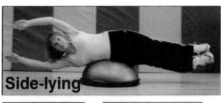

Side-lying

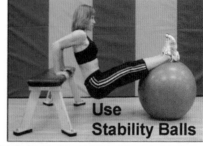

Use
Stability Balls

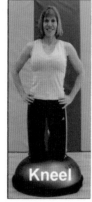

Kneel

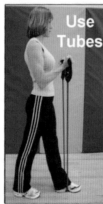

Use
Tubes

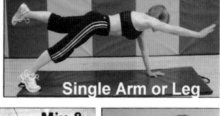

Single Arm or Leg

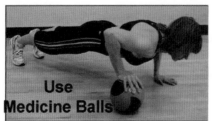

Use
Medicine Balls

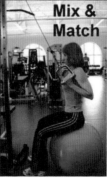

Mix &
Match

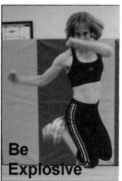

Be
Explosive

In the world of fitness, "CORE" is a magical word, and rightfully so, because without a strong core your limbs are useless. The core consists of all trunk muscles; glutes, hips, abs, and lower back. I hope by now you've gotten the message to engage your core by pulling your belly button back toward your spine at all times. Each time that you notice your stomach is sticking out, it is imperative that you pull it back in, especially when exercising. If you desire a firm strong midsection, understand that balance=belly. The more you utilize balance, the stronger your core muscles become.

Try standing on one foot to see how long you can hold your position. Now, extend one leg in front of you and hold this position for five seconds, then extend your leg to the side and hold for five seconds. Now, rotate your hips slightly, extend your leg behind you, and hold position for five seconds. Switch your feet and repeat the same movements. Did you do better on your right foot, left foot, or are you equally wobbly on both? Repeat these movements with your belly button pulled back toward your spine. You will notice it is much easier when your core muscles are engaged. To make balancing more challenging, repeat the same balance movements with your eyes closed. You will find it becomes very difficult. It is the job of your eyes to help you maintain balance by leveling your body with the horizon. While it is wise to always look straight ahead when balancing or performing exercises, you can progress some exercises by performing them with your eyes closed.

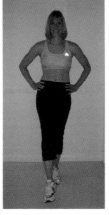 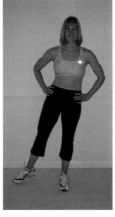 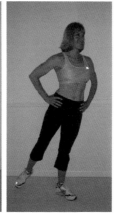

Your resistance-training program must include core and balance exercises. Good news! Core exercises can be performed every day. In order to maintain balance, your core must engage and recruit muscles. The more muscles you use, the more calories you will burn. If your goal is hypertrophy, do your bicep curls while sitting on a bench; but if your goal includes working on your core, then do your bicep curls while standing on one foot. This will force your body to maintain good form and prevent cheating, while exercising your muscles from head to toe. If you require your body to balance as it performs many of your exercises or tasks, you will work your core muscles more often, reduce your risk of falling, and save precious time, as well. For example, if you are on the phone at home, don't just stand there; do balance exercises. Balance pods, foam rollers, DynaDiscs®, and balance boards are all exercise tools designed to make your workouts more challenging. My personal favorite is the BOSU®. It is a fantastic tool for developing better balance and provides a more challenging workout while working your core muscles the entire time you are using it! I recommend that you choose at least one exercise for your lower back, glute, hip, obliques, and abdominals, performed in this order.

If you enjoy a particular sport or recreational activity, choose exercises that will enhance your skills. I am including some of the most popular activities among executives. If your favorite activity is among them, choose one or more of the exercises recommended and add them to your first resistance-training program. If not, you can find more exercises relevant to your sport or recreational activity on the Internet.

Running:

Triceps: prone extensions, rope cable extensions, reverse grip extensions

Back: face pulls, rear delt pulls, rows, superman crisscross

Abdominals: cable rotations, med ball ax chops, bicycle, windmills

Lats: straight bar and single arm pullovers, med ball pullovers

Hips: hello dollies, side-lying hip abduction, prone scissors

Soccer:

Legs: split lunge jumps, step-ups, lateral jumps, jump land and stick, squats

Hips: lateral jumps, hello dollies

Abdominals: med ball chops, hip thrusts, reverse crunches, figure eights

Triceps: overhead extensions

Golf:

Shoulder: PNF, external rotation, upright row

Abdominals: low cable chops, cable rotation, med ball chops, bicycles

Legs: med ball lunges with rotation, quad sets

Bicep and Forearm: reverse curls

Tricep and Forearm: reverse grip tricep extensions

Back: face pulls, thoracic extensions

Tennis:

Shoulder: PNF, external rotation, rear lateral raise, lateral raises

Hips: lateral jumps, hello dollies, side lying hip abduction

Legs: power step-ups, quad sets

Bicep and Forearm: reverse curls

Tricep and Forearm: reverse grip extensions, prone extensions

Softball:

Quadriceps: squats, single-leg squats, squat jumps, tuck jumps

Hamstrings and Glutes: lunges, split squat jumps, reverse bridges

Hips: side-lying hip abduction

Core: planks, med ball chops, ball scissors, windmills

Shoulders: alternating press, shrugs, PNF, external rotation

Lats: bent-over rows

Tricep: overhead extensions, skull crushers

Bicep: single-leg curls, hammer curls

Swimming:

Lats: pullovers, pull downs

Back: face pulls, superman crisscrosses, skydivers

Legs: squat jumps, tuck jumps, quad sets

Abdominal: med ball chops, cable rotation, bicycles, leg and arm press

Tricep: prone extensions, rear lateral raises, overhead extensions

Shoulders: PNF, external rotation, alternating shoulder press, sword draw

Basketball:

Legs: squats, quad sets, reverse bridges; squat, lateral, and tuck jumps

Hips: hello dollies, lateral jumps, side-lying hip abduction

Abdominal: med ball chops, v-sits on bench, figure eights

Tricep: prone extensions, reverse grip extensions

Bicep: barbell curl plus, reverse curls

Back: functional rows, rows

Shoulders: upright rows

Cycling:

Back: face pulls, rear delt pulls, thoracic extensions

Hips: hello dollies, side-lying hip abduction, prone scissors

Legs: split lunge jumps, power step-ups, tuck jumps, jump land and stick

Abdominal: med ball chops, planks, v-sits on bench, straight leg bicycles

Hiking:

Back: rows, functional rows, face pulls, superman crisscrosses

Tricep: prone extensions

Hip and Glute: prone scissors, ball glute raises

Legs: power step-ups, quad sets, reverse bridges, offset squats

Abdominals: v-sits on bench, leg and arm press, planks

Before you select the first resistance-training exercises for your exercise routine, you need to refer to the information that you have documented on your PAR-Q. Keep in mind that these exercises will be selected based on your self postural assessment. These targeted muscles are currently weak, so go easy on yourself. With each repetition you will get stronger.

Observation	Possible Imbalance(s)	Recommended Exercise(s)
Knees bow out	Glute muscles are weak & tight & hamstrings are tight	Ball Squat or Ball Bridge
Knees turn in	Glute muscles are weak and adductors are tight	Ball Squats
		Ball Bridges
		Hello Dollies
		Side Lying Hip Abduction
Rounded back with butt tucking under	Glutes and hips are weak	Prone Scissors
		Sky Divers
		Back Extensions
		Superman Crisscrosses
Hips shift	Glutes, transverse abdominis, and lower back muscles are weak	Ball Squats
		Single Leg Balances
		Single Leg Squats
Head falls forward	Spinal alignment is off	Chin Retractions
Hands fall forward	Upper back muscles are weak and pec muscles are tight	Rows
		Face pulls
Heels raise off floor; toes turn out	Calf muscles are weak and tight	Single Leg Balances
		Single Leg Squats
		Single Leg Calf Raises
Arched back with butt sticking out	Glute, hip and abdominal stabilizers weak	Floor Bridges
		Ball Bridges
		Ball Crunches

Once these exercises have been selected, add exercises that will help you become pain free, followed by exercises relevant to your sport, recreational activity, or hobby. Fill in any blank spaces with exercises you simply enjoy or would like to try. Now you have a workout program good for the next four to five weeks. It is designed specifically for you. Now you are training smarter, not harder.

Chapter Seven: Avoiding the Grim Reaper
Top threats to executive health

Our bodies were designed to eat, sleep, and reproduce. Yet for some reason, we have developed eating habits that are harmful to our bodies, many of us barely get enough sleep, and most fail to get the minimum daily required exercise that our body requires to stay healthy. As for reproduction, we excel. But we teach our children lifestyle habits that are detrimental to their health and hasten their deaths. A 2007 health study revealed that for the first time in American history, parents will outlive their children. I was stunned by this news, but quickly realized that I shouldn't have been. I know that the level of obesity among adults and children is out of control. My older clients are actually in better health than my clients who are 30 and younger.

If your job requires six-plus hours of sitting, high levels of daily stress, long commutes, even longer work hours and business travel, and you are not physically taking care of yourself, you may actually be sprinting toward the Grim Reaper. Assuming you would like to have a higher-quality and longer life, I recommend that you write down your priorities immediately and make **YOU** your first entry.

Is it hard telling yourself you don't have time to get a healthy snack or exercise, or tell your children you don't have time to play, or tell your spouse you would love to take that walk but you just have too much work to do? Imagine how hard it would be to hear a doctor tell you that you have a chronic disease or terminal illness; especially when you know deep down inside that you may have been able to prevent it. Imagine telling that same news to your loved ones.

Now that I have your attention, consider the following habits that will help keep the Grim Reaper at bay:

1. Sleep six to eight hours each night.
2. Take the time to eat breakfast!
3. Pre-pack healthy snacks and keep them in your car, office, and briefcase.
4. Don't stuff and don't starve! Eat three meals and two snacks every day.

5. Use a nine-inch plate for your meals.

6. Portion control your food! No single item should be bigger than a tennis ball.

7. Eat fruits and vegetables from a rainbow of colors.

8. Do not eat within two hours of your bedtime.

9. Avoid fast food, trans fats, and high-fructose corn syrup.

10. Limit liquid calories. Eliminate sodas, and consume plenty of water.

11. Take a multivitamin every day.

12. Stretch every day.

13. Exercise a minimum of 30 minutes, five days per week.

14. See your doctor for age-related health checks.

15. Know what stresses you and develop coping skills for those stressors.

People who exercise actually burn more calories while sleeping than non-exercisers do. An exercised body spends all night burning calories building and repairing muscles. Muscle burns 50 calories per pound, while fat burns only three. The more muscle you have, the more calories you burn. A winning combination is a good night's sleep and a body with a good muscle to fat ratio.

When you sleep your brain organizes the skills you learned during the day and strengthens nerves that help your memory. This gives you mental energy necessary to concentrate and master complex tasks the next day. People who don't get enough sleep increase their risk of heart disease, stroke, viral infections, diabetes, and obesity. Sleep deprivation elevates the levels of cortisol in the body. Cortisol is a stress hormone that is linked to obesity. In any case, who needs more stress hormones!

If you are following instructions, you didn't eat two hours before bed last night. Your body was able to focus on repairing your muscles and energizing your brain, instead of spending the night digesting a bowl of ice cream. You've had a good night's sleep and you haven't eaten in 10 to 12 hours. It's time to break-the-fast and jump start your metabolism. Keep in mind that skipping breakfast is linked to obesity. This is a great time to take your multivitamin. I take Centrum®

Silver®. Researchers at Berkeley have discovered that taking a multivitamin helps prevent DNA damage that causes cancer.

Hopefully, you are now, drinking water, tea, and coffee; and limiting juices and sodas loaded with sugar. I know you like your sodas and diet sodas, but they have no nutritional value whatsoever. Even worse, sodas have been recently linked to metabolic syndrome, obesity, kidney disease, and osteoporosis. Metabolic syndrome is a combination of several cardiovascular risk factors, including high blood pressure, high cholesterol, abdominal obesity and insulin resistance, resulting in diabetes. Some research has indicated that one can of soda per day may add up to 15 pounds a year, and it is estimated that the average American consumes 56 gallons of soda each year. It is a major contributor to our country's growing obesity problem. And if that isn't enough to convince you to give up sodas, according to the National Osteoporosis Foundation, the phosphates in soda may interfere with calcium absorption. Many orthopedic specialists agree with this data. Osteoporosis is a silent killer. It is responsible for millions of hip fractures, which are now the leading cause of death in elderly people. Do you really want to take the risk of being that person who fell and couldn't get up?

We all have stress from time to time, but chronic stress is a contributing factor to heart-related conditions, headaches, and chronic pain. Stress destroys our body from the inside out. You do not have control over some stress, so it is imperative that you do manage what stress you can control, and develop coping skills to deal with uncontrollable stresses. It is crucial to your overall health. First, you must identify what pushes your stress buttons. Then discover what de-stresses you and make it a habit. Try to adopt a positive attitude, laugh, exercise, take a nap, and learn to breathe. Breathing techniques are an efficient and fast way to get control of your stress and calm you down. The best advice I was ever given concerning stress was to "serve myself a beverage and then let it serve me." One of my favorite pleasures is to sit with a warm beverage in the winter or a cold beverage in the summer and drink it in complete silence. I urge you to try it sometime. It may work for you, as well.

20 Minute Stress Reliever

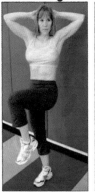
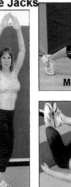
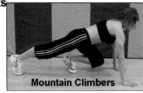

Mountain Climbers

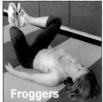

Froggers

Steam Engines: 30 seconds
Side Jumping Jacks: 1 minute
Mountain Climbers: 30 seconds
Flings: 1 minute
Mountain Climbers: 30 seconds
Overhead Squats: 20 reps
Pushups (your choice): 20 reps
Sky Divers: 15 reps 3 sec holds
Leg and Arm Press: 15 reps
Supine Floor Dips: 20 reps
Floor Bridges: 15 reps
Sidewinders: (alternate sides) 20 reps
Froggers: 60 reps
Hold Plank: 60 seconds
Repeat

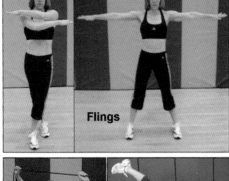

Flings

Supine Floor Dips

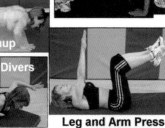

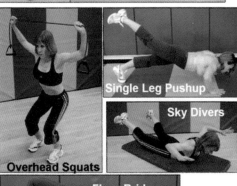

Single Leg Pushup

Sky Divers

Sidewinders

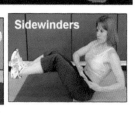

Overhead Squats

Leg and Arm Press

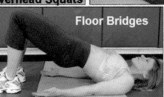

Floor Bridges

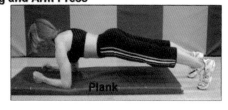

Plank

High cholesterol, high blood pressure, and other heart-related illnesses are a commonality among Americans. The majority of treatment plans use medications, rather than diet and exercise, to keep these conditions under control. My uncle is a respected pharmacist, so I am not suggesting that some people aren't in need of medications. I am suggesting however, that there is a greater demand for these medications simply because people are not eating a proper diet or performing minimal exercise. This becomes evident when many people are taken off cholesterol and blood pressure meds soon after their new diet and exercise program takes effect. Anyway, taking medications shouldn't be seen as a "quick fix." The patient should still be required to eat a proper diet and exercise while taking the medication. You may as well make diet and exercise a part of your life and, possibly, avoid ever needing supplemental medication. You will not be able to find a single piece of research that states, "Eating healthy foods and performing moderate exercise are bad for people with high blood pressure and high cholesterol." So, plan your food intake each day and get movin'!

Say this out loud three times: "Travel will not disrupt my diet and exercise goals." Now, click your heels together three times and wish you were home. You didn't really expect to be home, did you?

Travel is a part of our personal and, for many, our professional lives. We are a very mobile society. I have found that learning to incorporate healthy habits into a traveling lifestyle is very difficult.

A traveler loses control over food choices by restaurant availability, by being restricted to what is on a menu, and by the inability to prepare the food. A traveler cannot control traffic, weather, or airport delays. A traveler is as likely to arrive much later than expected as to arrive on time. In addition, each time a time zone is passed; it becomes more and more difficult to get enough sleep. It is not unusual for a traveler to be too emotionally or physically drained to even think about exercise. In the airport terminal a traveler must maneuver through a minefield of giant cinnamon buns, colossal muffins, and small doughnuts packing a huge saturated fat explosion. If traveling by car, the choices are usually grease, grease, and more grease.

What can you control if you travel? You can control your snacks by pre-packing unsalted nuts, raw vegetables, fresh fruit, dried fruit, cereal, pretzels, or hard-boiled eggs, just to name a few. Trade your soda and juices for water. Water is not only healthier but it will help you stay hydrated, especially when flying. Go topless (and I don't mean take your shirt off) by avoiding harmful condiments that add calories. Instead of mayo, go for mustard. Top a salad with a light or fat-free dressing. Order your food baked, grilled or broiled instead of fried, and stick to turkey, chicken, and fish. Do not eat bread unless you can get whole-wheat or whole-grain. If you hit the coffee shop, order tea or coffee (tall, non-fat, and no whip), and avoid muffins large enough to feed a family of four, or anything named "mocha caramel" or "frappuccino."

If you have glitches in your day that reduce or eliminate the time you allotted for exercise, the "No Gym Required" workout is a great alternative. It takes only 30 minutes to complete and requires no equipment. This workout can be done virtually anywhere. Even if you don't have 30 minutes, at least stretch after you shower and perform a few body-weight exercises to relieve your back from a long day of sitting and to regain circulation in your legs. This should help you sleep better.

In addition, if you are going to cross time zones and can sleep while traveling, by all means, do so. It would also be wise to take a nap the day after you arrive, to help you catch up on your zzzz's.

"No Gym Required" Workout

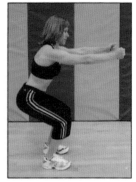
Squats

Body Weight Squats: 20 reps
Alternating Lunges: 20 reps
Alternating Side Lunges: 20 reps
Overhead Claps, Forward Circles, Backward Circles:10 each
Static Push (arms straight fingers point to ceiling): 10 seconds
Floor Tricep Humps (each arm): 20 reps
Squat Thrusts: 15 reps
Mountain Climbers: 30 seconds
Diagonal Jumps Right: 45 seconds
Prone Scissors: 1 minute
Ice Skaters: 45 seconds Calf Raises: 15 seconds
Flutter Kicks: 50 seconds then hold for 15 seconds
Clap Jacks: 90 seconds
Dive Bombers: 10 reps
Jump, Land and Stick: 10 reps right 10 reps left
Double Crunches: 30 seconds
Toe Reach Crunches: 30 seconds
Diagonal Jumps Left: 45 seconds
Superman Crisscross: 1 minute
Squat Flings: 30 seconds

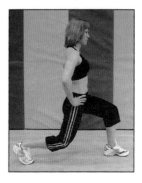
Lunges

Hold stretches for 30 seconds each:
Toothpick Stretch (elongate your body)
Hamstring with Ankle Rotation right/left
IT Band Stretch right/left
Knees to Chest
Lying Glute
Lying Extensions
Cat/Camel
Childs Pose

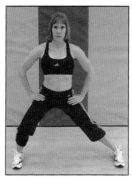
Side Lunges

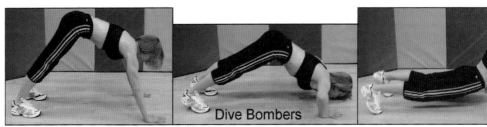
Dive Bombers

Traci Trainer

Jump, Land & Stick

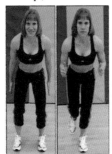

Clap Jacks

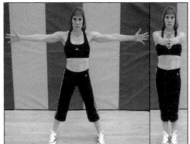

Superman Crisscross

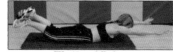

Flutter Kicks

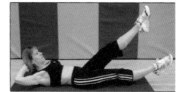

Diagonal Jumps

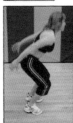

Double Crunches

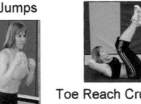

Floor Tricep Humps

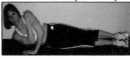

Toe Reach Crunches

Squat Flings

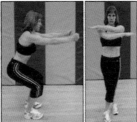

Prone Scissors

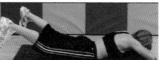

Mountain Climbers

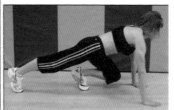

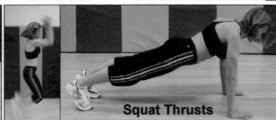

Squat Thrusts

Cat Camel Stretch

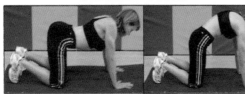

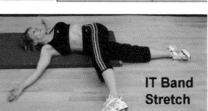

IT Band Stretch

Lying Extension

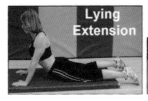

Childs Pose

Knees to Chest

Lying Glute

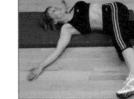

Chapter Eight: Did you know?

Health nuggets that could change your life

-Drink a half glass of warm water, take half a regular aspirin, and drink the remaining half glass of water. It can decrease your risk of getting colon, esophageal, prostate, ovarian, and breast cancer by 40 percent. Discuss with your doctor if this is right for you!

- If you are under age 60, get 800 IU of vitamin D daily; over age 60, get 1,000 IU daily, or expose your skin to 20 minutes of sunlight daily. Vitamin D may decrease your risk of cancer because it is toxic to cancer cells. Deficiency of folate, which is part of the B-complex vitamins, is linked to cancer. Foods like spinach, tomatoes, and orange juice contain folate, but you probably need to supplement 400 micrograms in order to reduce your risk of cancer.

-Oolong tea contains polyphenols, which help control body fat by improving the metabolism of nutritional fat.

-Taking two daily doses of chia seed, 20 grams each, lowers blood pressure and the risk of heart problems.

-People who sleep less than six hours per night increase their risk of viral infections, heart disease, and stroke by 50 percent.

-Taking a 30-minute nap may increase productivity and reduce your risk of a fatal heart attack by 37 percent.

-Melatonin, available in health food stores, helps reset your body clock when having travel-related sleep issues.

-More men than women die of osteoporosis finds a new review in the *Canadian Medical Association Journal*. One contributor is lack of sleep leading to low levels of testosterone. Men with less testosterone are more prone to bone loss. Do not be the one in eight men who will develop the bone-thinning silent killer. Of those men who have osteoporosis, 40 percent are more likely than women to die of hip fracture complications.

-Fast food restaurants are obesity minefields. Eating just one double quarter pounder with cheese per week contains enough calories to add nearly six pounds a year to your body. A latte and cake at a coffee shop contains more than 900 calories.

-Drinking two cups of coffee daily reduces your risk of liver cancer by 43 percent.

-Regularly drinking just half a can of soda raises your risk of diabetes. Researcher's tracked people who drank six ounces of soda daily and found they are 67 percent more likely to have Type -2 Diabetes than non-soda drinkers.

-Sit in a reclined posture. It causes less spinal pressure than sitting upright or hunching forward.

-Plyometric exercises, such as jumping, use all of your large lower-body muscles and raise your metabolism. They help firm up and shape your butt, hips and thighs, while strengthening your legs at the same time.

-The more muscles you engage when performing an exercise, the more calories you will burn. By combining upper- and lower-body exercises, your body is forced to work harder in order to balance and stabilize itself. Also, when your body is required to use numerous muscles while engaging its core; it elevates your heart rate, burning more calories and saving your overall workout time.

-Interval training improves fat burn in men and women. Train intensely when trying to lose body fat because you'll burn more calories during the workout as well as burn more calories after the exercise session is over.

-During exercise, muscles need more oxygen and produce more lactic acid which is eventually converted to carbon dioxide. Breathe in via your nose for three counts and exhale via your mouth for three counts throughout the day at work, as well as when exercising.

-According to a recent article in *Men's Health* magazine; 64 percent of active adults under age 45 suffer from joint pain. Choosing functional exercises that mimic your daily lifestyle can reduce your risk of joint injury. For example, fit exercises into your routine that will help you lift a heavy suitcase in the airport, get a briefcase out of your backseat, or sprint to the gate where your flight is about to take off without you.

-According to the American Heart Association 90 percent of adults between ages 55 and 65 are at risk for hypertension.

-If you thought the 10-minute routine was hard imagine jumping rope for one hour and seventeen minutes just to burn off two slices of Pizza Hut stuffed crust cheese pizza.

-The number one junk food sold during 2007 in the United States was soda. The FDA portion size is eight ounces but the average amount of a single serving sold in restaurants is 19.9 ounces.

-According to a recent article in *Men's Health magazine*; the average weight gained by sedentary people who ate two fast-food meals a day for one month was 14.1 pounds.

<u>Exercises</u>

Traci Trainer

Chest

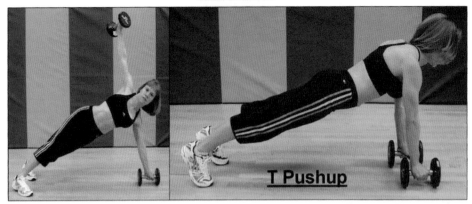

T Pushup

Remember: draw in abs, keep feet hip-width apart, back flat, lift with obliques!

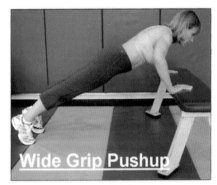

Wide Grip Pushup

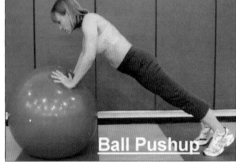

Ball Pushup

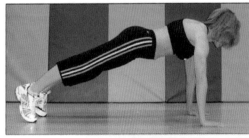

Make it harder by taking your knee to your opposite elbow!

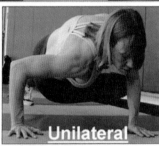

Unilateral

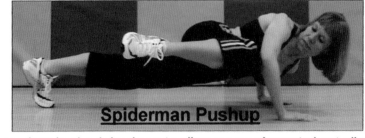

Spiderman Pushup

Remember: draw in abs, bring knee to elbow as you lower to bent elbow position

Traci Trainer

Back

Stability Ball Row

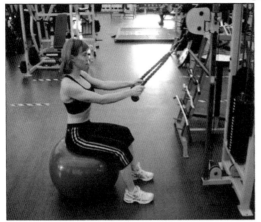 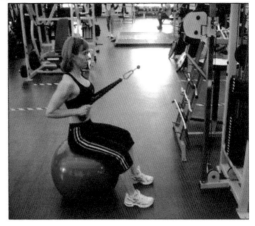

Remember: keep feet hip width apart, toes pointed straight ahead, draw in abs while pulling ropes into a row using your back

Squat to Row with BOSU

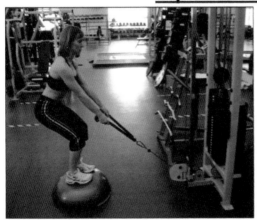 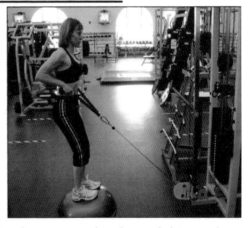

Remember: draw in abs for stability, keep your back straight, push through heels while pulling ropes into a row using your back

Prone Flys

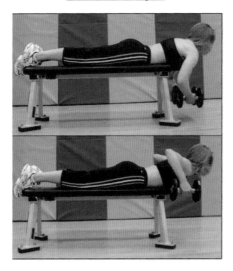

Remember:
*keep head in line with spine
*draw in abs
*do not raise chest off bench
*stay in pain free range of motion

Lying Extensions

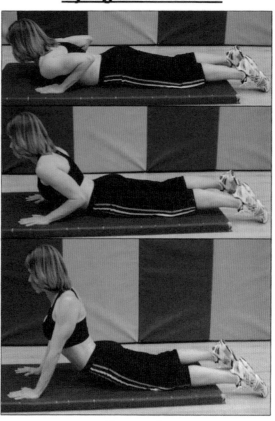

Remember:
*keep shoulders down
*stay in pain free range of motion
*3 second hold when elevated

Rear Delt Pulls

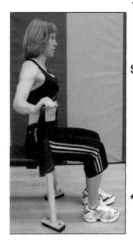

Remember:
*start with arms
straight in front of
you extended
*draw in abs
*keep shoulders
back and down
*keep elbows
slightly bent
*do not use neck!

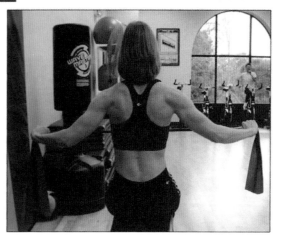

82

Ball Bridge Progression

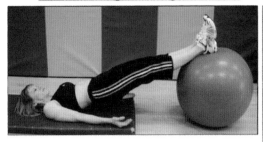

Feet Flat on Ball

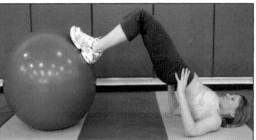

Advanced

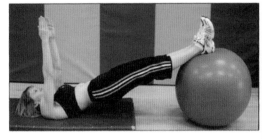

Advanced

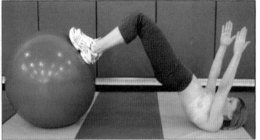

Single Leg

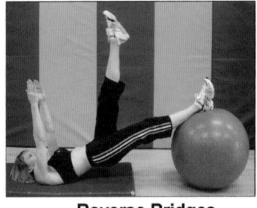

Single Leg

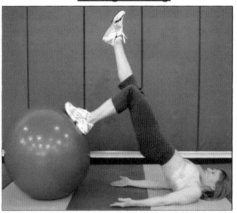

Reverse Bridges

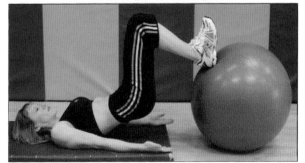

Remember:
*draw in abs
*squeeze glutes lifting pelvis
into bridge
*point toes toward head

Traci Trainer

Lat Pullover   Single Arm

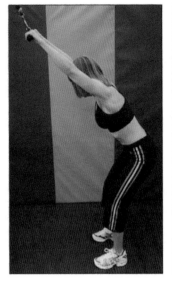 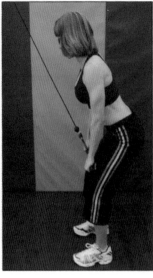 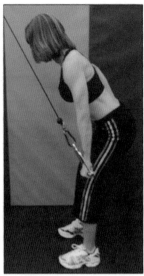

Lat Pull Downs

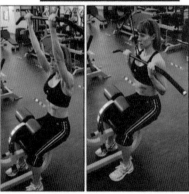

Remember:
*draw in abs
*keep feet hip width apart
*toes pointed straight ahead
*engage lat before pulling down
*set shoulders back and down
*do not elevate your shoulders
*exercise should not be felt in your neck!

Med Ball Lat Pullover

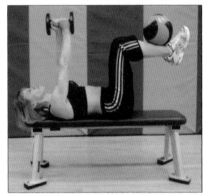 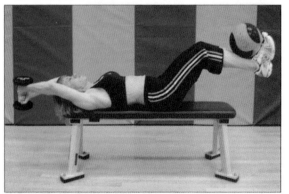

Remember: draw in abs, keep back flat against bench, and engage lat before pulling.

Traci Trainer

Ball Back Extensions

Remember:
*draw in abs for balance
*keep feet together
*drop legs as far as possible
*raise legs together
*squeeze butt at top
holding for 2 seconds

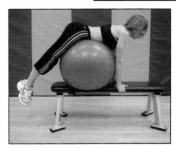 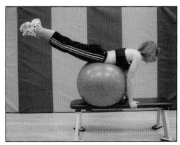

Ball Bridge with Butt Drop

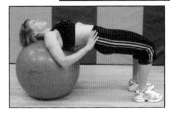 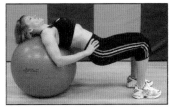

Remember:
*drawn in abs for balance
*keep feet hip-width apart
* toes point straight ahead
*raise hips into bridge by
squeezing your glute
*hold bridge for 2 seconds

Thoracic Extensions

Remember:
*drawn in abs
*lift upper body into an extension
*stay in a pain free range of motion
*do not push on your head or neck

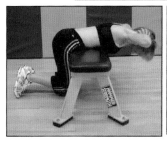 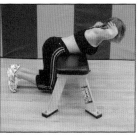

Back Extensions   Remember: squeeze glute taking 4 seconds to raise

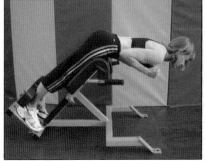 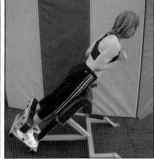 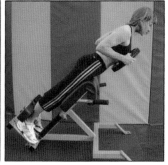

Traci Trainer

85

Superman Crisscross

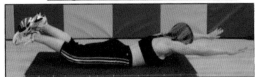

Remember:
*draw in abs
*keep head in line with spine
*cross feet over then under

Sky Divers

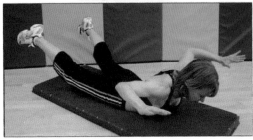

Remember:
*draw in abs
*from resting position lift up
into sky diving pose
*hold position for 3 seconds

Opposite Arm/Leg Extension

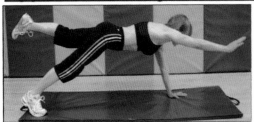

Remember:
*draw in abs
*lift leg first then opposite arm
*hold position for 3-5 seconds
*regress to knees if needed

Floor Bridges

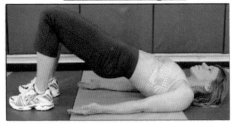

Remember:
*draw in abs
*feet hip width apart
*toes pointed straight ahead
*squeeze glute lifting into a bridge
*movement should be slow and
controlled
*if knees go out hold a
rolled up towel between them

Rope Cable Face Pull

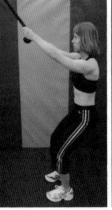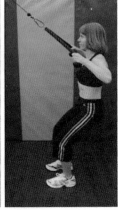

Remember:
*draw in abs
*keep back flat
*feet hip width apart
*toes pointed straight ahead
*keep movement out of neck
*pull out and back
*squeezing shoulder blades together

Seated Stack Rows

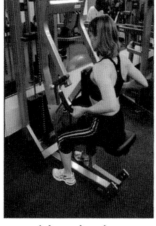

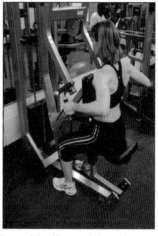

Remember:
*feet hip width apart
*toes pointed straight ahead

*draw in abs
*back straight

*head in line with spine
*do not jut neck forward
*do not elevate shoulders

Barbell Rows

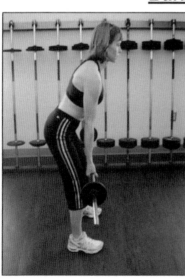

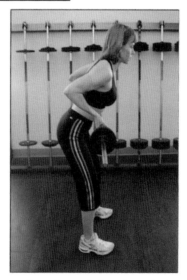

Remember: feet hip width apart, toes pointed straight ahead, back straight, draw in abs, keep head in line with spine, pull bar into a row using your back, do not elevate your shoulders or use your neck to execute movement

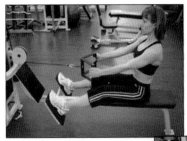

V Grip Cable
Row

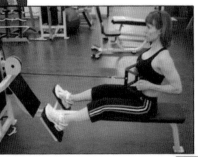

Single Arm
Row

Remember:
*keep feet hip width apart
*toes pointed straight ahead
*knees slightly bent
*draw in abs
*pull with your back not your bicep
*move in a pain free range of motion
*no jerky motions
*do not rock back and forth

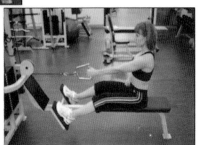

Single Arm Cable Row with Rotation

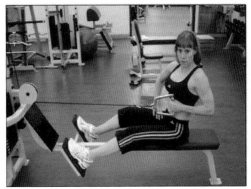 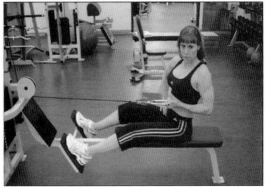

Traci Trainer

Prone Tricep Extensions

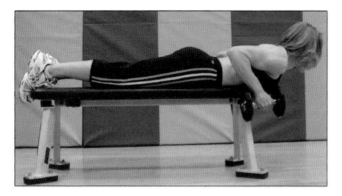

Tricep

Remember:
*draw in abs
*keep head in line with spine
*keep upper body stationary
*do not let elbows drop
*kick weights straight back

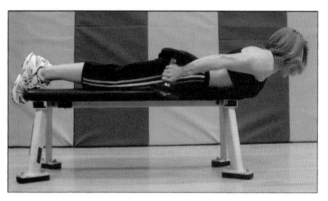

Barbell Skull Crusher

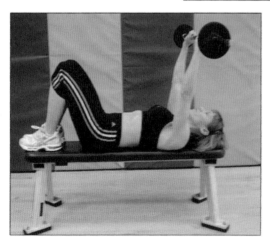 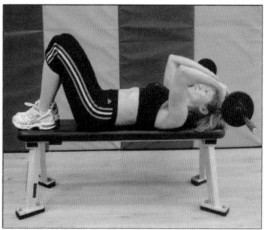

Remember: draw in abs, use a towel for lumbar support if needed, do not let elbows move, move elbow to wrist only, dumbbells can also be used

Overhead Tricep Extension

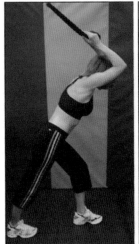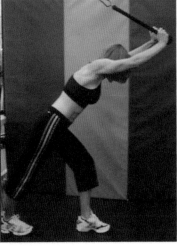

Remember:
*draw in abs
*stagger your stance
*keep upper body stationary
*keep elbows next to ears when extending arms

Reverse Grip Tricep Extension

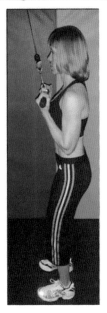

Remember:
*draw in abs
*shoulders and elbows
in line with hips
*do not rock

Rope Cable Tricep Extension

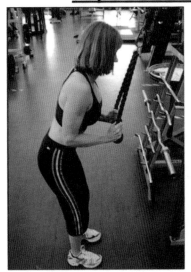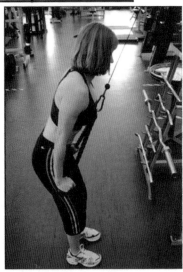

Remember: draw in abs, feet hip width apart,
toes pointed straight ahead, keep elbows and
shoulders in line with hips, elbows super glued to
sides, do not rock, keep upper body stationary

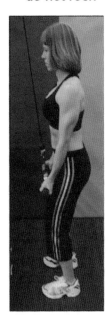

Single Leg Curls

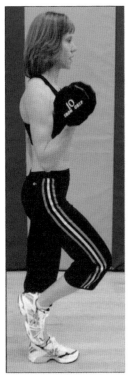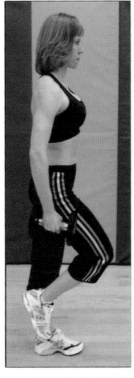

Bicep

Remember:
*draw in abs
*keep shoulders back and down
*alternate arms with each curl
*keep elbows slightly bent
*arms out to side
*never lock out elbows
*keep toes close enough to floor
to tap down

Hammer Curls

Remember:
*draw in abs
*squeeze glutes
like sitting on rocks
*keep shoulders back
and down
*raise arms up and
over shoulders
*do not take
weights past ears
*elbows slightly bent
*movement should
be slow and
controlled
*take 4 seconds to
lift and lower weights

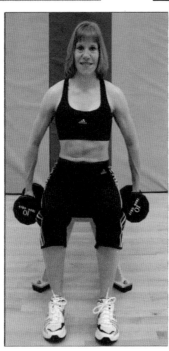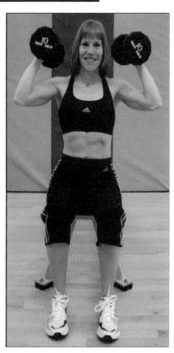

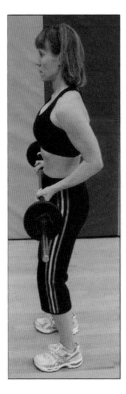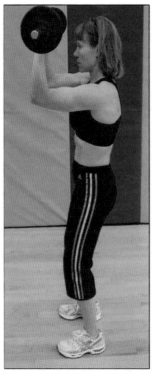

Barbell Curl Plus

Remember:
*draw in abs
*feet hip width apart
*toes pointed straight ahead
*knees slightly bent
*do not elevate shoulders
*move at the shoulder
*do not move elbow to wrist
*using your abs and
bicep push dumbbell
out and up
*take 4 seconds to
lift and lower barbell
*you can also use
a cable machine

Reverse Curl

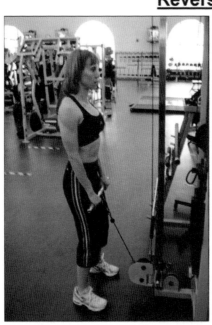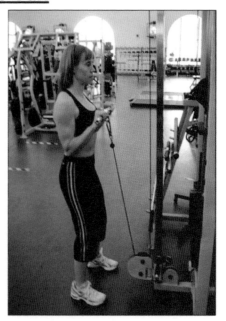

Remember: feet hip width apart, toes pointed straight ahead,
draw in abs, keep elbows tight to sides, do not let wrists bend

Traci Trainer

Shoulder

Side Lying External Rotation

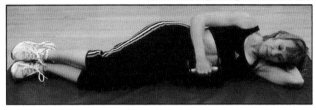

Remember:
*draw in abs
*rest your head
*use light weight
*move in pain free range of motion

PNF

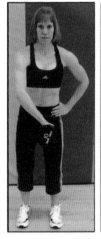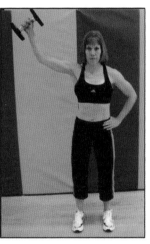

Remember:
*draw in abs
*feet hip width apart
*toes pointed straight ahead
*move in pain free range of motion
*use light weight
*keep elbow slightly bent

Elbow Pulls

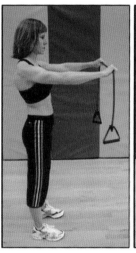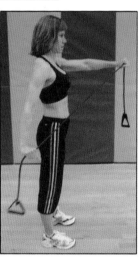

Remember:
*draw in abs
*feet hip width apart
*toes pointed ahead
*elbows and knees slightly bent
*pull tube back and down
*do not elevate shoulder into neck

Upright Row

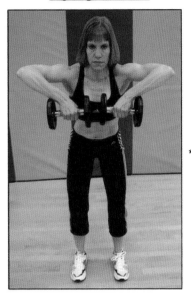

Lateral Raise

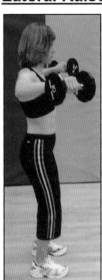

Remember:
*draw in abs
*feet hip width apart
*toes pointed straight ahead
*knees flexed
*keep elbows slightly
in front of you for upright row
*keep elbows bent 90 degrees
while performing
lateral raises
*lateral raises can also be
performed seated
*do not allow movement
to be felt in your neck

Bent Over Rear Lateral Raise

Remember:
*draw in abs
*feet hip width apart
*toes pointed straight ahead
*keep head in line with spine
* keep upper body stationary
*use back of shoulder to pull
weight behind you
*move in
pain free range of motion

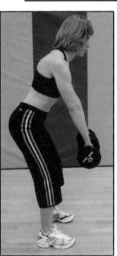
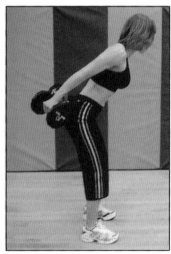

Alternating Shoulder Press

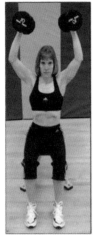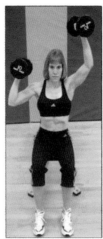

Remember:
*draw in abs
*feet hip width apart toes pointed straight ahead
*squeeze glutes like you're sitting on rocks
*hold arms slightly in front of ear
*leave one arm up at all times
*move other arm in pumping motion

Squat to Front Raise

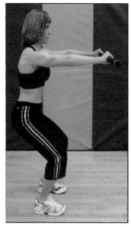

Remember:
*draw in abs
*do not let your knees go over your toes
*raise bar shoulder height
while performing a squat
*movement should be slow and controlled

Pulsed Lateral Raises

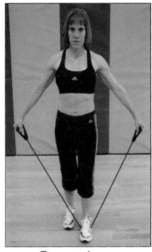

Remember:
*set shoulders back and down
*raise handles to point of tension
*keep tension while pulsing

Sword Draw

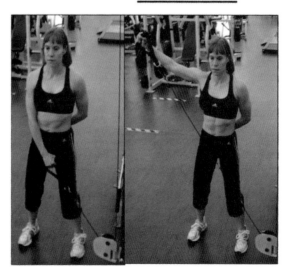

Remember: move in pain free range of motion but do not twist at the waist

Functional Rows

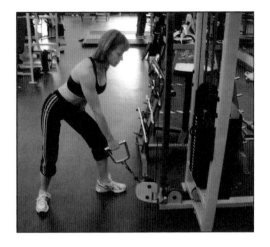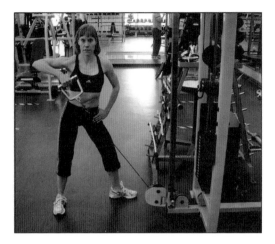

Remember: keep knees bent, feet in "L" shape so knees are in line with toes, pull handle using abs and shoulder girdle into an elbow strike

Behind the Back Shrugs

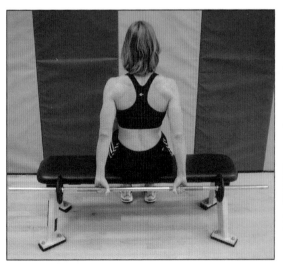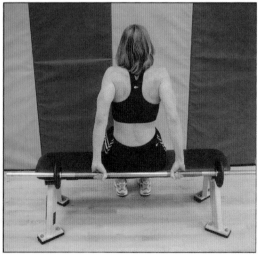

Remember: draw in abs, keep feet hip width apart, toes pointed straight ahead

Core

Hello Dollies

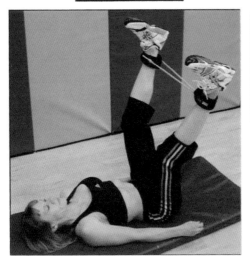

Side Lying Hip Abduction

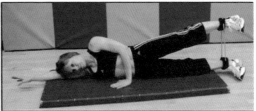

Remember:
*draw in abs
*rest ear on arm
* raise leg to point of tension
*pulse at point of tension
*keep toes pointed straight

Dirty Dogs

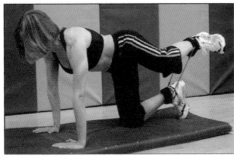

Remember: lift and lower leg keeping legs bent 90 degrees

Prone Scissors

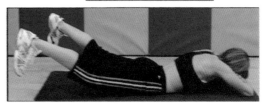

Remember:
*rest forehead on arms
*point toes toward floor
*open and close legs

2Ball Glute Raise

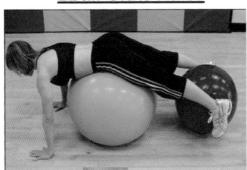

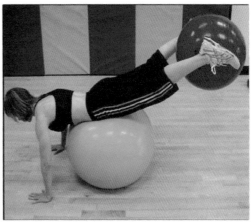

Remember: draw in abs, squeeze glutes to lift legs

V-Ups

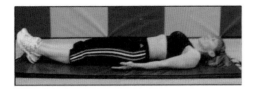
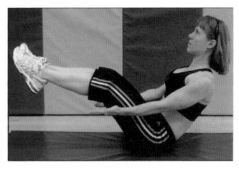

Figure 4 Crunches

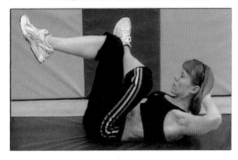

Hundreds

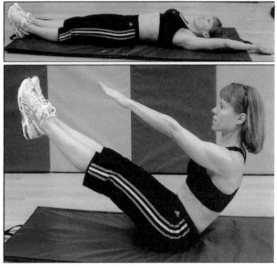

Remember:
*draw in abs
*keep shoulders back and down
*pull up using abs
*keep back straight
*keep elbows wide
*do not pull on your neck or head

V-Sit Oblique Crunches

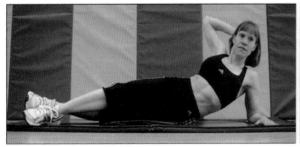
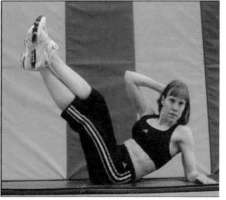

Traci Trainer

BOSU Supine Balance

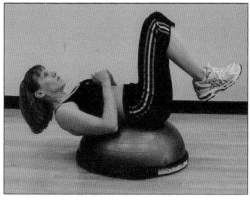

BOSU Bicycle

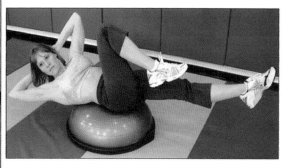

BOSU Hip Abduction

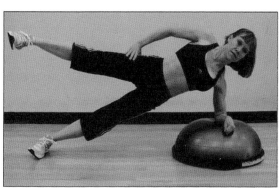

Opposite Arm/Leg Balance

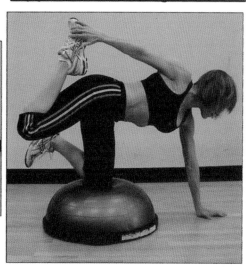

BOSU Crunch

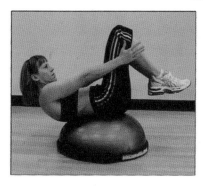
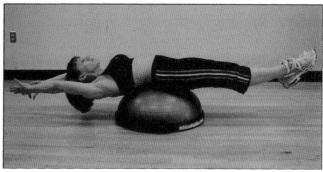

Traci Trainer

BOSU Sky Diver

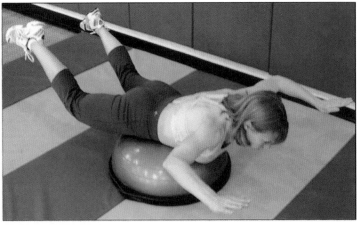

BOSU Burpee

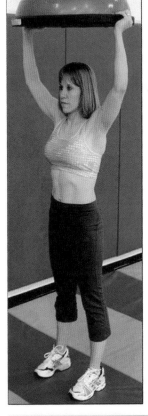

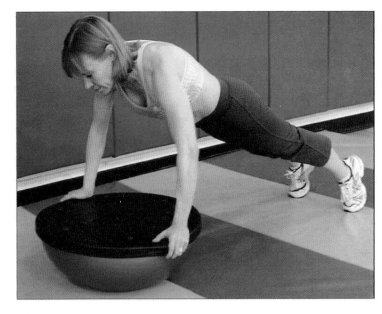

BOSU Oblique Crunches

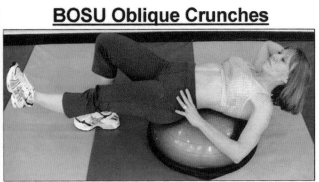

Reverse Crunch

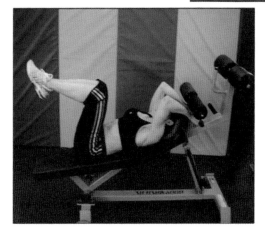 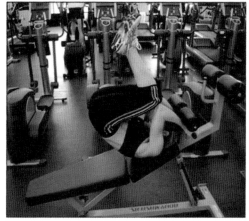

Reverse Crunch with Rotation

Hip Thrust

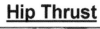

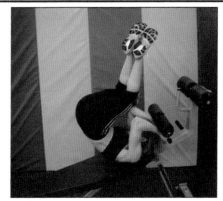 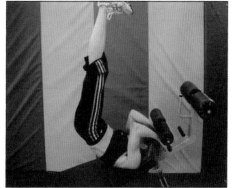

Reverse Crunch with Med Ball

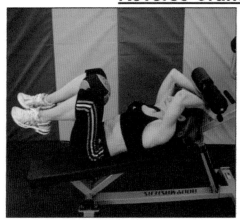 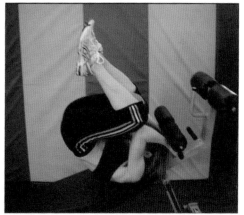

Remember: stop your butt from hitting the bench (within two inches)
then pull up using your lower abs until reps are complete

Russian Twist

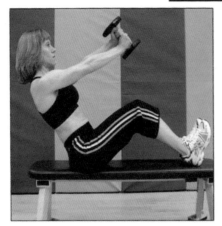 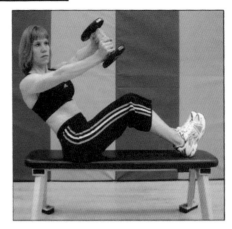

Remember: draw in abs, keep shoulders back and down, keep feet and knees together, toes pointed toward head, twist to each side keeping shoulders square, correct form if necessary when returning to center position

Leg and Arm Press

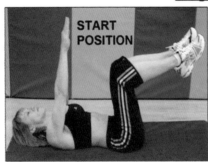

START POSITION

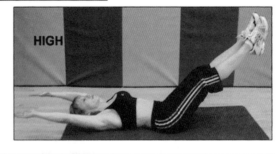

HIGH

Remember:
*draw in abs
*use towel for lumbar support if needed
*movement should be slow and controlled
*breathe

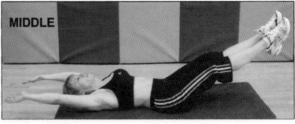

MIDDLE

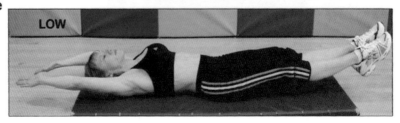

LOW

Traci Trainer

Ball Scissors

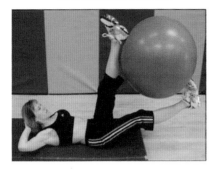

Figure 8's

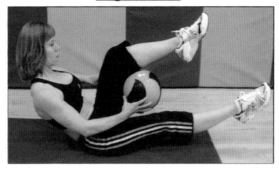

V sits on Bench

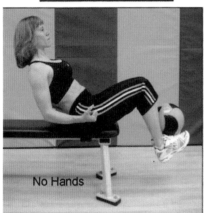

No Hands

Remember for all exercises on this page:
*draw in abs
*keep back flat
*when lying down keep shoulders off the floor
*keep a slow pace
*do not use momentum to execute movement
*keep elbows wide
*do not pull on your head or neck

Bicycles

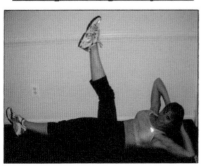

Straight Leg Bicycles

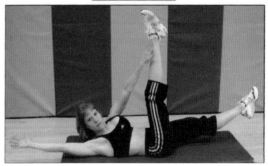

Windmills

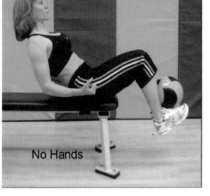

Ball Crunches

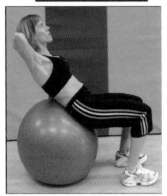

Remember:
*draw in abs
*feet hip width apart toes pointed straight ahead
*knees bent 90 degrees
*look at 45 degree angle
*keep elbows wide while performing crunch

Med Ball Chops

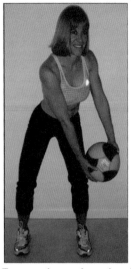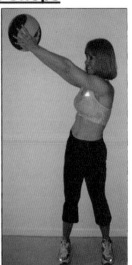

Remember: draw in abs, keep arms straight, lift ball using obliques as if throwing a pail of water over your shoulder, keep both feet on the floor during movement

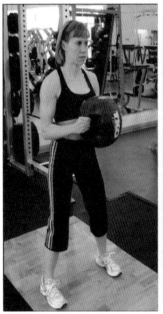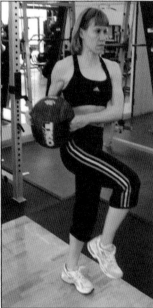

Med Ball Ax Chops

Remember:
*draw in abs
*feet hip width apart
*toes straight ahead
*do not elevate shoulders
*keep shoulders squared to front while twisting med ball to the side of your hip

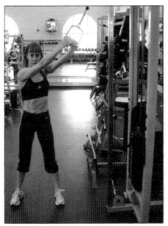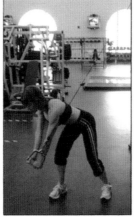

High Cable Chop

Remember:
*draw in and pull with abs
*keep arms straight
*perform at slow pace
*move in pain free
range of motion

Cable
Rotation

Remember:
*draw in and pull with abs
*keep arms straight
*perform at slow pace
*move in pain free
range of motion
*do not allow feet to lift
off floor

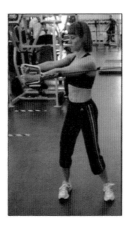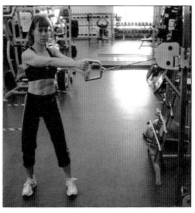

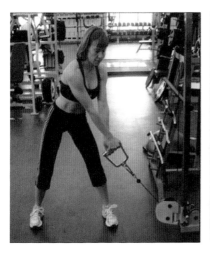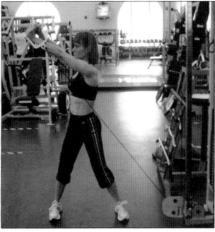

Low Cable Chop

Legs

Offset Squat

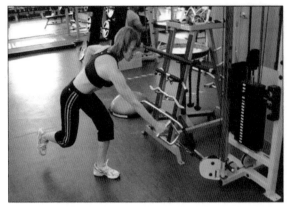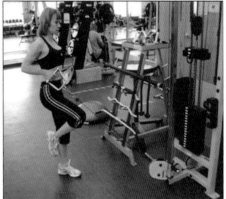

Remember: draw in abs while pushing through your heel pull with your back

Serratus Pulls

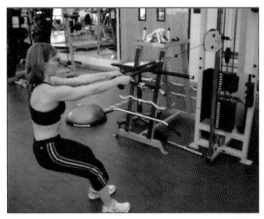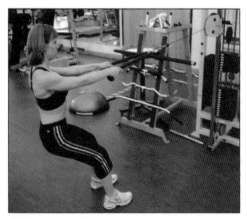

Remember:
*draw in abs
*keep back and arms straight
*knees slightly bent
*pull under your arm
*do not lean back

Med Ball Rotation Lunges

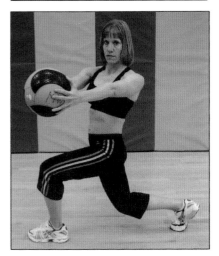

Quad Sets

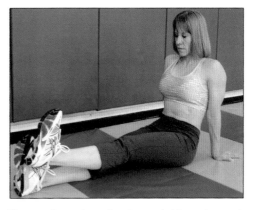

Remember: draw in abs, point toes toward face, hold leg six inches off floor for 10 seconds

Remember: draw in abs, keep arms straight, do not allow knee to go over toe, twist holding ball to the same side you lunge

Single Leg Calf Raises

Ball Squats

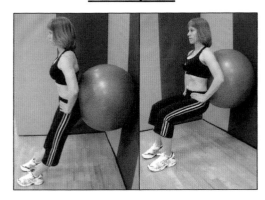

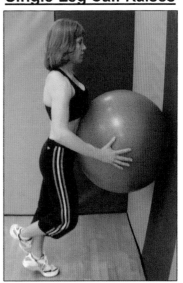

Remember: draw in abs, push thru heels, squeezing glute to come up!

Remember: draw in abs, lift and lower heel, ensure your foot stays pointed straight ahead

Power Step Ups

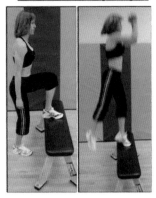

Remember:
*draw in abs
*push off leg
on floor
*explode up

Split Lunge Jumps

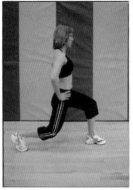 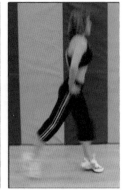

Remember: keep torso straight, draw in abs

Lateral Jumps

Remember:
*tuck your laces
*draw in abs
*form before speed

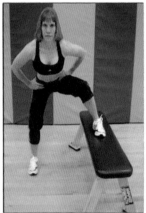 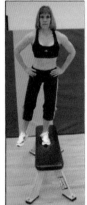 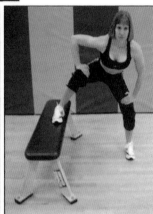

Jump Land & Stick

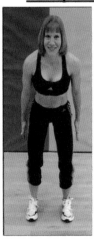 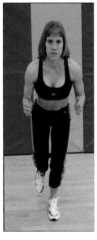

Remember:
*start jump
with both
feet
*land on
one foot
straight
ahead

Hip Twist Jumps

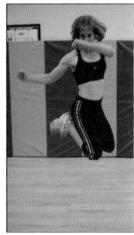

Remember:
*feet must
land in
original
position
with feet
pointed
straight
ahead

Bibliography

Alter, Michael J., <u>Sport Stretch</u>. United States: Human Kinetics, 1998.

Chu, Donald A., Ph.D. <u>Jumping Into Plyometrics</u>. United States: Human Kinetics, 1998.

DiNubile, Nicholas A., M.D., <u>Frame Work</u>. United States: Holtzbrinck, 2005.

Holt, David. "Exercise Decreases Osteoporosis and Bone Fractures." <u>Running Dialogue Today</u>, June 1997.

Mercola, Joseph, Dr., and Droege, Rachael. "The Real Dangers of Soda to You and Your Children." <u>Take Control of Your Health,</u> July 2003.

Jackowski, Edward J., <u>Hold It! You're exercising wrong</u>. New York: Simon & Schuster, 1995.

Jemmett, Rick. <u>Spinal Stabilization: The New Science of Back Pain</u>, 2nd Edition. Nova Scotia: Novant Health Publishing Limited, 2003.

Marano, Hara Estroff. "The Rewards of Shut-Eye." <u>Psychology Today</u>. April 2003.

Mc Kenzie, Robin. <u>Treat Your Own Back</u>. New Zealand: Spinal Publications, 1981.

McKenzie, Robin. <u>Treat Your Own Neck</u>. New Zealand: Spinal Publications, 1983.

National Academy of Sports Medicine. <u>Optimum Performance Training for the Health and Fitness Professional, 2nd Edition</u>. United States: National Academy of Sports Medicine, 2004.

O'Connor, Anahad. "Too much cola can cause kidney problems." <u>New York Times,</u> February 2008.

Oz, Mehemt C., M.D., and Roizen, Michael F., M.D. <u>You On A Diet</u>. New York: Simon & Schuster, 2006.

Oz, Mehmet C., M.D., and Roizen, Michael F., M.D. <u>You Staying Young</u>. New York: Simon & Schuster, 2007.

Paroe, Lee. <u>Power Posture.</u> Vancouver: Apple Publishing Company Ltd., 2002.

Presidents and Fellows of Harvard College. "Breakfast and your health." <u>Harvard Publications,</u> June 2006.

Radcliffe, James C. <u>Functional Training For Athletes At All Levels</u>. California: Ulysses Press, 2007.

Reuters. "Soda linked to increased metabolic risk." <u>Reuters,</u> July 2007.

Thieme, Trevor. "Iron Out the Kinks." <u>Best Life,</u> March 2007.

Index

A

B

C

D
Diabetes, 11, 69, 70, 77
Dips, 59
Dirty Dogs, 97
Dorsiflex, 39

E
Elbow Pulls, 93
Erector Spinae Stretch, 44
External Rotation, 93

F
Facepulls, 86
Figure Eights, 103
Figure Four Crunches, 98
Flexibility, 27, 28, 32, 37, 38
Floor Bridges, 86
Forearm Stretch, 47
Frozen Shoulder, 33
Functional Rows, 96

G
Gait, 13, 26
Golf, 20, 33, 45, 46, 65

H
Hammer Curls, 91
Hamstrings, 27-30, 33, 37, 45, 46, 65
Heart Disease, 11, 69
Heel Spurs, 25, 26
Hello Dollies, 97
Herniated Disc, 32
Hip Flexor Stretch, 30
Hip Thrusts, 101
Hip Twist Jumps, 108
Hundreds, 98

I
Iliotibial Syndrome, 28
Interval Training, 50, 54, 55
IT Band Stretch, 28, 47

J
Jump, Land and Stick, 108

K

L
Lateral Jumps, 108
Lateral Raises, 94, 95
Lat Pull Downs, 84
Lat Pull Overs, 84
Lat Stretch, 47

Made in the USA